Housing and home
in later life

RETHINKING AGEING SERIES

Series editor: Brian Gearing
School of Health and Social Welfare
The Open University

'Open University Press' *Rethinking Ageing* series has yet to put a foot wrong and its latest additions are well up to standard . . . The series is fast becoming an essential part of the canon. If I ever win the lottery, I shall treat myself to the full set in hardback . . .'

Nursing Times

Current and forthcoming titles:
Miriam Bernard: **Promoting health in old age**
Simon Biggs *et al.*: **Elder abuse in perspective**
Ken Blakemore and Margaret Boneham: **Age, race and ethnicity**
Julia Bond and Lynne Corner: **Quality of life and older people**
Joanna Bornat (ed.): **Reminiscence reviewed**
Bill Bytheway: **Ageism**
Anthony Chiva and David Stears (eds): **Promoting the health of older people**
Maureen Crane: **Understanding older homeless people**
Mike Hepworth: **Stories of ageing**
Frances Heywood *et al.*: **Housing and home in later life**
Beverley Hughes: **Older people and community care**
Tom Kitwood: **Dementia reconsidered**
Eric Midwinter: **Pensioned off**
Sheila Peace *et al.*: **Re-evaluating residential care**
Thomas Scharf *et al.*: **Ageing in rural Europe**
Moyra Sidell: **Health in old age**
Robert Slater: **The psychology of growing old**
John A. Vincent: **Politics, power and old age**
Alan Walker and Tony Maltby: **Ageing Europe**
Alan Walker and Gerhard Naegele (eds): **The politics of old age in Europe**

Housing and home in later life

Kintiner

FRANCES HEYWOOD,
CHRISTINE OLDMAN and
ROBIN MEANS

OPEN UNIVERSITY PRESS
Buckingham • Philadelphia

Open University Press
Celtic Court
22 Ballmoor
Buckingham
MK18 1XW

email: enquiries@openup.co.uk
world wide web: www.openup.co.uk

and

325 Chestnut Street
Philadelphia, PA 19106, uSA

First Published 2002

A catalogue record of this book is available from the British Library

ISBN 0 335 20169 5 (pb)   0 335 20170 9 (hb)

Library of Congress Cataloging-in-Publication Data
Heywood, Frances.
    Housing and home in later life/Frances Heywood, Christine Oldman,
    Robin Means.
      p.   cm. – (Rethinking ageing series)
    Includes bibliographical references and index.
    ISBN 0–335–20170–9 – ISBN 0–335–20169–5 (pbk)
    1. Aged–Dwellings–Great Britain. 2. Aged–Housing–Great Britain.
    3. Aged–Services for–Great Britain. 4. Home ownership–Great Britain.
    I. Oldman, Christine. II. Means, Robin. III. Title. IV. Series.

HD7287.92.G7 H49 2001
363.5'946'0941–dc21

                                                    2001021411

Typeset by Type Study, Scarborough
Printed in Great Britain by
St Edmundsbury Press, Bury St Edmunds, Suffolk

In memory of Lyn Harrison

Contents

List of boxes and tables   viii
Series editor's preface   ix
Acknowledgements   xii

1   Housing and home in later life: an introduction   1

Part I   Reviewing the issues   19
2   Theories, assumptions and policies   21
3   The housing issues of old age: different perspectives   40
4   Housing, health and community care   61

Part II   Reporting empirical studies   75
5   To move or not to move: housing decisions in later life   77
6   Maintaining independence: repair, adaptations and design   96
7   Living in communal settings   118
8   Working together in the interests of older people?   137
9   Conclusions   155

References   169
Index   181

List of boxes and tables

Box 1.1   More life experience   6
Box 1.2   Fear of extreme old age   10
Box 3.1   The experience of home carers, 1999   54
Box 3.2   Some practical housing issues presented from the
           perspective of older people   55
Box 5.1   The HOOP questionnaire   91

Table 1.1   Population changes and percentages of older people
             in the UK, 1901–97   13
Table 1.2   Changes in living arrangements of older people,
             1891–1994   14
Table 3.1   Illustration of government perspective on services
             to older people   44
Table 4.1   Percentage of older people reporting long-standing
             illness   69
Table 5.1   Factors pushing older people to move   86
Table 5.2   Some attractions of moving to alternative
             accommodation   88
Table 5.3   Some factors pulling people to stay in their current
             homes   89
Table 7.1   Key characteristics of institutions and home   120
Table 8.1   Dimensions of user involvement   139
Table 8.2   'Need to know' good practice checklist   152

Series editor's preface

In the second year of the new century, we are now some 17 books into the 'Rethinking Ageing' series and it seems appropriate to review our original aims. The series was planned in the early 1990s, following the rapid growth in ageing populations in Britain and other countires that led to a dramatic increase in academic and professional interest in gerontology. In the 1970s and 1980s there was a steady increase in the publication of research studies which attempted to define and describe the characteristics and needs of older people. There were also a small number of theoretical attempts to reconceptualize the meaning of old age and to explore new ways in which we could think about ageing. By the 1990s, however, a palpable gap had emerged between what was known about ageing by gerontologists and the very limited amount of information which was readily available and accessible to the growing number of people with a professional or personal interest in old age. The 'Rethinking Ageing' series was conceived as a response to that 'knowledge gap'.

The first book to be published in the new series was *Age, Race and Ethnicity* by Ken Blakemore and Margaret Boneham. In the series editor's preface I set out the main aim of the 'Rethinking Ageing' series: To bridge the knowledge gap with books which would focus on a topic of current concern or interest in ageing (ageism, elder abuse, health in later life, dementia, etc.). Accordingly, each book would address two fundamental questions: What is known about this topic? And, what are the policy and practice implications of this knowledge? We wanted authors to provide a readable and stimulating review of current knowledge, but also to *rethink* their subject area by developing their own ideas in the light of their particular research and experience. We also believed it was essential that the books should be both scholarly *and* written in clear, non-technical language that would appeal equally to a broad range of students, academics and professionals with a common interest in ageing and age care.

The books published so far in the series have ranged broadly in subject matter – from ageism to reminiscence to community care to pensions to residential care. We have been very pleased that the response from individual readers and reviewers has been extremely positive towards almost all of the titles. The success of the series appears therefore to justify its original aims. But how different is the national situation in gerontology more than ten years on? And do we now need to adopt a different approach? The most striking change is that, today, age and ageing are prominent topics in media and government policy debates. This reflects a new awareness in the media and among politicians of the demographic situation – by 2007 there will be more people over pensionable age than there will be children.[1] Paradoxically, however, the number of social gerontology courses is actually decreasing.[2] Why this is so is not entirely clear, but it is probably related to the difficulties which social and health care workers face in securing the time and funding to attend courses. Alongside this is the pressure on course providers to give priority to the short-term training needs of care staff through short, problem-focused modules. Only a few gerontology courses are based around an in-depth and truly integrated curriculum, one that draws upon the very many different academic disciplines and professional perspectives which contribute to our knowledge and understanding of ageing.

There is more interest in ageing and old age than when we started the 'Rethinking Ageing' series, and this persuades us that there is likely to be a continuing need for the serious but accessible, topic-based books in ageing that it offers. The uncertainties about the future of gerontological education reinforce this view. However, having now addressed many of the established, mainstream topics, we feel it is time to extend its subject-matter to include emerging topics in ageing, as well as those whose importance have yet to be widely appreciated. Among the first books to reflect this policy were Maureen Crane's *Understanding Older Homeless People* and John Vincent's *Politics, Power and Old Age*. More recently, Mike Hepworth's *Stories of Ageing* was the first book by an author based in the UK to explore the potential of literary fiction as a gerontological resource.

Most older people live and die in ordinary housing in the community. This is one impetus behind *Housing and Home in Later Life* by Frances Heywood, Christine Oldman and Robin Means. As well as filling a gap in the series, it makes a major contribution to the literature on ageing in a neglected topic area. The authors are respected members of a network of knowledge and practice relating to housing policy and older people in the UK. In writing this book they were able to draw on their own recent research in the field, and on research where they have been involved as advisors. Interaction with professionals and with older people on postgraduate, professional and continuing education courses and seminars have enriched this research knowledge.

All three authors are strongly committed to user centred research on housing and older people. One of the major issues that runs through their book is how housing and housing-related policies might change for the better if the views of older people were seriously heeded. This question of how older people wish to live is examined in the light of recent research.

The book also considers what policy of community care would promote the health and well being of older people living out their lives in their own homes. It looks at the extent to which the housing element of community care is being addressed and also looks specifically at the changing community care role of sheltered housing and at residential/nursing homes as a place of residence for older people. Housing policies are considered too in the light of theories on the meaning of home in later life and theoretical perspectives on old age.

This is both a broad and inclusive book which rethinks its subject. It is a particularly welcome addition to the 'Rethinking Ageing' series. In future, we hope to continue to rethink ageing by revisiting topics already dealt with (via second editions of existing titles) and by finding new titles which can extend the subject matter of the series.

Brian Gearing
School of Health and Social Welfare
The Opening University

Notes

1 *Guardian*, 29 May 1999.
2 Bernard, M *et al.* in *Generations Review*, Vol. 9, No. 3, September 1999.

Acknowledgements

The authors wish to thank especially the following people: Randall Smith, Reader, and Professor Martin Boddy at the University of Bristol for their patience and encouragement; Professor Mary Maynard at the University of York for her support for Chapter 2; Professors Peter Malpass, Rodney Lowe, Pat Thane and Harry Henry for information, publications and guidance on the historical analysis in Chapter 1; Malcolm Hornsby, historian and bookseller, for advice and the most generous loan and supply of rare books; John Galvin and the Elderly Accommodation Counsel for permission to use the material in Chapter 5; Bernadette Cox from the University of the West of England, Lynne Lonsdale, secretary at the Centre for Housing Policy, University of York, who prepared the final manuscript with such cheerfulness, and support staff at the School for Policy Studies, including Clare Biddlecome and Angela Torrington; our respective families and friends, who have endured so much from us while we have been working on this book and, finally, the editorial staff at Open University Press for their patience in waiting for it. Each of us would also like to acknowledge the help we have received from the others.

The book is richer for the inputs of these various people, but needless to say, any errors contained in it are our own.

1

Housing and home in later life: an introduction

Purpose of the book

Why write a book about the housing issues of later life? How can this be justified when, within the text, we argue that the habit of classifying older people as a group separate from other adults is, in many contexts, not rational? In fact, this habit may be as pernicious as the separation in other societies of people into 'Jew' and 'Aryan' or 'Black', 'White' and 'Coloured'. The analogy is useful though, because in those societies there were real differences between the groups identified but they were not the differences that were originally described and then used to justify discrimination. It is our task in this book, therefore, to consider four things:

- the 'genuinely' distinctive characteristics of later life
- the implications of these characteristics for social and housing policies
- the provision that currently exists
- the changes in thinking that are needed if policies are to be based on the first two points above rather than, as now, on a 'medical' model of old age.

The purpose of the book is both to describe the here and now and to challenge ourselves and the reader to rethink assumptions and the policies that are based on them. At the heart of all policies supporting people to live and thrive into old age lies the concept of home. Yet there is a vacuum where policies concerning housing issues should be and such policies as exist are, we shall argue, ageist. Individuals who reject them are left to find what solutions to their living arrangements they can. Despite all the rhetoric of community care, the neglect of issues relating to housing and the home is widespread. All three of us have a commitment to see the issue of housing and home in later life rethought so that the diverse needs and preferences of a group who constitute around one-quarter of the population are more adequately addressed. To different degrees, we have all been involved in both social policy research and practice. It is the academic discipline of social policy which underpins the book but we also, we hope helpfully, employ a historical and sociological perspective.

This book is concerned with housing and social policy relating to older people. However, in contrast to other discussions, for example Mackintosh *et al.* (1990) and Oldman (1990), policies are not the dependent variable. The central focus, rather, is on older people and their domestic environments: their homes and their housing. The book is primarily about housing and home in later life in the UK; however, from time to time we refer to the experiences of other countries.

The purpose of this chapter is to set the scene. It starts by defining terms: what is meant by 'later life', by 'housing' and by 'home'. 'Diversity and difference' are explored. A very brief overview of diversity *within* old age is presented followed by a discussion of some of the distinctive characteristics of later life that are to be borne in mind throughout the following chapters. Then follows a discussion of the historical roots of housing circumstance in later life. A historical perspective is enormously valuable in any exercise involving analysis of current policies. At the end of the chapter the current policy landscape which forms the backdrop to the rest of the book is introduced.

Definitions

Later life

Definitions of 'old age' and 'later life' are well known for being socially and culturally bound. Old age in Britain is still defined in terms of the official retirement age, although more and more people are leaving the working force early. At the present time 18.2 per cent of England's population is 'elderly', that is, over 65 if male, over 60 if female. We want our definition of 'later life' to be quite flexible. It needs, among other things, to be culturally sensitive. Britain is a multicultural society and within its varied cultures views will differ considerably. For some, retirement from paid work at 60 or 65 is the watershed, but people who started work as very young children in overseas countries and had hard lives ever since might feel they had earned a rest by the age of 45 or so. For male gypsies in Britain whose life expectancy at the end of the twentieth century was 55 (Hawes 1997), 'later life' must also begin earlier. In Vietnamese culture, grandparenthood marks entrance into the category of 'older people' but this would not be accepted universally. Some people see their youngest child leave home when they themselves are in their forties, and are able to begin a new phase of life. Other parents are still attending school events in their sixties. It is not unknown for people to be in receipt of both old age pension and child benefit. In general, however, 'later life' is defined by a combination of chronological age and life course experience. A person under 50 years old would not normally be included in the definition in Britain in the twenty-first century but there will be exceptions when life has aged people prematurely. Crane's (1999) discussion of homelessness and older people, also in this series, raises for the reader questions about the definition of 'old'. A lifetime of 'secure' accommodation, a roof over your head, however inadequate, unsuitable and unaffordable that accommodation may have been, is a quite different experience from a lifetime of insecure accommodation, a lifetime in and out of homelessness. Mortality and morbidity rates among homeless people are higher than for those who have a home. When does 'later life' begin for people whose life has mainly been characterized by homelessness? Definitions of old age could usefully employ a housing perspective.

'Later life' is not a euphemism for old age but a description of a phase that begins, arguably for most, around 50 and may then cover five decades of varied experience. But it is not adolescence, it is not young adulthood, it is not early middle age. It is the latter part of life, after a midpoint in terms of maximum expected life span has been reached. 'Old age' as we use it implies a greater age, beginning around 70. Extreme old age describes those who are 90 and over.

Housing

Housing is a physical structure within which a self-selected household lives. It is a place in which the basic human activities of sleeping, eating, washing, storage of possessions, social contact, recreation and care within the self-selected household take place. The word may also incorporate the attributes of the structure: its location, size, design, condition, accessibility, affordability, warmth and comfort. The word is also applied to a collection of such structures which includes the provision of facilities for shared use. The terms upon which housing is occupied (that is, its forms of tenure) will vary. They include owner occupation (freehold or leasehold, with or without a mortgage), renting from a council, private landlord or housing association (again with varying degrees of security) and membership of a housing cooperative.

Housing is the focal point for communication between the citizen and the state and the citizen and other people, an organic hub serviced by a range of professionals including postal workers, refuse collectors, meter readers and others, all necessary to its functioning as housing. As an active verb form, it can also imply the daily responsibilities of paying for, maintaining and managing the property, deciding who lives there and accepting the duties of paying, not just for the structure but for such consequent items as water, gas, electricity or council tax. For professionals, the verb also means the provision, management or maintenance of such structures and their surrounding environments. However, as we shall note throughout the book, these services, whether they come from social housing landlords or private agencies, in a direct way affect only a minority of the older population.

Home

Housing is a word imbued with technical meaning. Home denotes the existential and the experiential. Home is where domestic lives are played out. However, as Chapman and Hockey (1999) note, the discipline of sociology has been relatively silent on the subject of home. Certainly, within social gerontology (the study of the social aspects of ageing) there has been little interest in it. There is a body of literature from within housing studies on the 'meaning' of home in general and in later life in particular but this (it will be shown in Chapter 2) is fairly narrowly construed.

Home is a myriad of things: it is a set of relationships with others, it is a statement about self-image and identity, it is a place of privacy and refuge, it is a set of memories, it is social and physical space and so on (Benjamin and Stea 1995). There is a widely held assumption that in later life the home assumes a central importance that it may not necessarily have had in the past, that it provides for older people their main focus in life. It is one of the purposes of this book to subject this sort of conventional wisdom to some scrutiny.

Diversity in later life

The point has been well made by many writers in the literature on ageing that it is absurd to impute any homogeneity to later life. Any reassessment of the housing and social policy environment must recognize and respond to the diversity within later life. On any number of dimensions there is enormous diversity. Here we note just five that are particularly relevant to the concerns of this book.

Chronological age

Later life spans a period of some 40 years or so. In terms of factors such as life experience, generational effects and health profiles, there are enormous differences. Housing policies aimed generally at the 'elderly' seem likely to fail unless they recognize that the 60-year-old home-owner in many ways is likely to be a very different person from the 85-year-old home-owner. The 'baby boomers' (those born in the two post-1945 population bulges) quite clearly differ from those older people born before the Second World War (Evandrou 1997).

Income and wealth

Diversity relating to income and wealth is of crucial importance to the arguments that we shall present. Although the end of paid employment represents for many a decline in economic fortunes, the income inequalities of younger life continue and, in some cases, deepen in later life (Hancock 1997). Early retirement policies have hit some older people hard in financial terms. Only 50 per cent of household heads aged 55–64 are in full-time employment. Although some have been happy to leave the workforce, some have not. Since 1981 the gap between the richest and poorest pensioners has grown. Taking the case of single pensioners, the poorest 20 per cent had an average weekly income of £68.00 with the richest 20 per cent having £205 (Department of Social Security (DSS) 1998a). Moreover, there is gender diversity.

Two-thirds of men over pensionable age have non-state pensions, but three-quarters of women are not in this position (Ginn and Arber 1996). Tenure is an important indicator of financial diversity within old age. Tenure, income and disability are all closely related. Older people, living in different forms of rented housing, are poorer and unhealthier than those living in the owner-occupied sector, although there are considerable income disparities within the latter (Hancock 2000). Moreover, there is considerable diversity of housing wealth. Over one-third of all those over retirement age have no equity at all and there are wide variations around the mean level of equity held (Leather 1999). About 5 per cent of older owners are both income rich and equity rich, 40 per cent are income poor and equity rich and a similar proportion are neither rich nor poor as they fall into the middle income and equity bands. At the bottom of the distribution 15 per cent of older home-owners are both income and equity poor.

Ethnicity

As Blakemore and Boneham (1994) have noted, although the overwhelming majority of the older UK population is white, the differences in the needs and aspirations of older people from minority ethnic groups compared to those of the 'white' population need to be reflected in housing, health and social care policies. Policy makers need to note that besides clear differences between the majority white population and black and other minority older people, there is considerable diversity within the latter population. Diversity both between and within should be celebrated rather than 'ironed out' (Williams 1989). Policy makers need to heed that, while small numerically, at the start of the twenty-first century (3 per cent of minority ethnic people over 65), by 2020 there will be a significant increase in the older black and minority population (Patel 1999).

Housing status

Although the vast majority of the older population are 'housed', there is a far larger segment of that population than previously thought who are living in insecure accommodation or sleeping rough. Homeless acceptances (that is, accepted by local authorities as homeless because of 'vulnerability') relating to people over pensionable age are considered to be a serious underestimation of the numbers involved (Hawes 1997; Crane 1999).

Rural/urban

The majority of the older population live in urban or suburban settings. However, that significant group who live in the countryside are particularly unseen and unheard (Help the Aged 1992). For older people problems with access to services and appropriate housing can mean increasing isolation and loss of independence.

Difference

There is an inevitable tension running through this book. We argue that treating old age as a separate category serves to perpetuate the ageism that is so endemic in western society. On the other hand, for policies to be more inclusive and helpful there must be a recognition of those distinctive features of later life which have a bearing on home and housing.

Experience

Older people have not necessarily had more varied housing experience than younger people, for they may have lived a very long time – even all their lives – in one house and not visited very widely. They have, however, had more life experience (see Box 1.1). They have lived through more different eras and fashions, seen more policies (and governments) come and go and are more aware of long-term consequences. This experience also makes older people more sceptical of promises and guarantees, knowing how a situation that seems to be for ever may be overturned by some unforeseen event. Experience may also be the reason why older people are often tolerant and reluctant to complain. They have learnt not to expect too much, and they have also often learnt that complaining (even when invited) is likely to alienate service providers. This factor makes it necessary for professionals to be very cautious in interpreting housing satisfaction surveys carried out with older people.

Life achievement

One difference between a 25-year-old householder and a 75-year-old is 50 years of working and living. In housing terms, this may be reflected directly in the property, in work done to the home over many years, trees planted,

---

Box 1.1   More life experience

Early in the year 2000 a New Labour Member of Parliament (MP), parliamentary private secretary to a minister, was addressing a local Labour Party meeting. Among those present were a couple who had belonged to the party for over 60 years, both having joined in the 1930s. The MP told the gathering that the government had achieved 'more free prescriptions than ever before'. She did not seem either pleased or convinced when the older couple interrupted to say that when the National Health Service (NHS) was introduced *all* prescriptions (*and* teeth *and* glasses) were free. The long memories and long perspective of older people illustrate a characteristic of later life that younger politicians and professionals often ignore, because they are unaware of it.

furniture and carpets worked for and paid for, decorating and alterations, curtains lovingly (or painstakingly) made.

Dwellings are used by all age groups as a means of demonstrating achievement and status. Not everybody collects china or likes to display trophies, photographs or presents, but if people are inclined to do these things, they will have more when they are older. And if physical decline has enforced a less active lifestyle, the older person may take some consoling pleasure from the symbols of achievement that their home and its contents represent.

More leisure

If 'leisure' is defined as time when a person may choose what they do, most people have more of it in later life than they did when they were younger and had no choice but to go school or to work. In later life, some people continue in full-time paid employment because they want to, need to or are afraid to stop. Some exchange paid employment for unpaid employment caring for a parent, a spouse or other person who has become frail or ill, and find they have less leisure time than ever.

But for a good number of people there is at last a chance to make choices about the use of time: to do voluntary work, socialize, study or pursue a range of creative or recreational activities. However, leisure may become a burden rather than an opportunity. Leisure costs money. A key difference between older people and younger age cohorts lies in income levels. Nearly two-thirds of those over 70 are among the poorest 40 per cent of the population and the remainder are only half as likely as those in other age groups to be among the richest 40 per cent of the population (Royal Commission 1999).

In housing terms, the implications of increased leisure time are that people will spend far more time in their home – so that comfort, aesthetics and affordable warmth all become more important than they may have been in the past. Access to facilities or to transport to facilities become the key aspects of location. For couples the need to adjust to sharing the domestic space full time may be a problem and a place of escape – whether garden shed or small spare room cum sewing-room – crucial. Space to pursue interests or voluntary activities is another key housing implication.

Grandparenthood (or equivalent relations with a generation twice removed)

Grandparenthood, many older people would say, is one of the great privileges of later life. It is a joy no more understood or attainable by younger people than the glory of Homer in the original Greek can be by those who have not spend years studying to reach a point where they can read it. Because they are young, demanding and without preconceptions, grandchildren can be a powerful modernizing and revitalizing force in their grandparents' lives – pulling them away from their peer group towards the interests, tastes and expectations of a new generation. This is why so many people say that their grandchildren 'keep them young'. There is often a gentle conspiracy between grandparents and grandchildren against the intervening generation.

Grandparenthood can go on a very long time and extend to great-grandparenthood, so it is not possible to make an all-encompassing statement about its implications for housing, but there are some core points to be made.

Policy makers, we shall argue, see older people as isolated, solitary creatures requiring only minimal space. People with grandchildren (or great-nephews and nieces) will want them to be able to visit and, often, to stay. Both grandparents and great-grandparents may have cots and highchairs kept for such visits, and needing storage space. Sometimes, through divorce or death, or as a matter of child protection, the grandparents will give a child a home long term or permanently and will need the space to do so.

Within the Asian communities in Britain it is quite common to send a grandchild to live with grandparents in order to help them in old age. The child's parents may be only a few doors away, but the grandchild moves in to give the best possible support. Allocation policies in the public sector, based on narrow 'housing need' criteria, have militated against these kinds of customs in the established communities in Britain. In the United States the development of common interest developments (CIDs) with stringent lease conditions may similarly prevent this grandparent–grandchild bond by forbidding the residence on the estate of anyone under 50 (McKenzie 1994).

Finally, as grandparents and grandchildren both grow older, there may come a time when housing problems put the relationship at risk. If people are forced to use commodes or become smelly through not being able to bathe, pride and compassion may mean that older people will not want their grandchildren to have to cope with these things – and so will discourage contact if solutions cannot be found.

Declining health

One of the most obvious characteristics of later life that has a direct bearing on housing provision is the tendency to reduced mobility and agility caused by the diseases of old age. Osteoporosis, rheumatoid arthritis, diabetes, cardiovascular diseases and various problems associated with sensory impairment affect large numbers of people in later life. They make it generally harder for people to climb stairs, take a bath or carry out jobs in the house or garden. These changes may come on very gradually or suddenly without warning, as in the case of a stroke. How they affect people's ability to enjoy their home depends on the design of the home in the first place, and/or on the possibility of adaptation, both issues that are considered at length in later chapters because they are so fundamental.

In noting the changes in physical characteristics which are a feature of later life, the tendency to pathologize old age must be avoided. The various statistical data sources relating to morbidity and disability show that poor health and its consequences are not a universal experience. For example, although the proportions increase with age, only 30 per cent of those over 65 have trouble with steps and stairs and 77 per cent are 'independent' (Office for National Statistics (ONS) 1999b: 11).

Similarly, declining mental health has to be placed in context. 'Only' one in five of those over 80 or over will have some form of dementia (Lord Chancellor's Department 1997). However, for those who are afflicted and for their families the problem is real enough. We attempt at various points in the book to consider and explore housing and home in later life in the context of failing cognitive abilities. More common than dementia in its various forms and yet more neglected in terms of policies, provision and service delivery are other mental health problems such as depression, whose incidence is higher in later life than in younger life (Coleman 1994).

Likelihood of bereavement

If people are in a couple, or live with a sibling, the chances are that one will die before the other and one will be left bereaved and alone in a home they formerly shared. Apart from the grief this can cause, there are immediate housing consequences as so many costs will continue unaltered while income may be halved. If the partner who has died was the only driver, the survivor may also be left very isolated.

Awareness of mortality

People become increasingly aware of the approach of death as they get older. Such awareness is difficult to avoid as friends and family begin to die, but reactions may be different. Some face up to death and begin to prepare for it; others work frenetically to defy or deny it. It makes its impact either way.

In housing terms, those who face up to death may be inclined to stop spending money on their home, on the grounds that it would be a waste of money and the house is good enough to 'see them out'. Having made such a decision, they may live twenty years longer, with serious consequences in terms of growing disrepair. Many will be concerned to leave a legacy to their children and may try for instance to give the house to them seven years before death in order to avoid inheritance tax. The focus as death approaches shifts from oneself to one's descendants, and passing on the house becomes like the grandchildren, an opportunity to achieve some continuity or legacy of yourself, even after death, by helping your offspring to thrive.

Fear of extreme old age

It may be true that many people (young and old) are more afraid of extreme old age 'sans teeth, sans eyes, sans taste, sans everything' than they are of death itself (see Box 1.2). In Britain, in contrast to some other European countries, there is widespread fear of the residential home, of the relinquishing of householder status. This characteristic of later life is hugely important, as it is part of what drives people to remain in their own home against all odds, and to put up with discomfort, cold, loneliness and worry rather than surrender to what is commonly regarded as the last resort.

Box 1.2   Fear of extreme old age

In *Gulliver's Travels*, first published in 1726, there is a description of the Struldbruggs, a subspecies of people in the land of Luggnagg who, unlike the normal inhabitants, grow old but do not die. Before he meets the Struldbruggs, Gulliver imagines the glory of being immortal, but he is rapidly disabused. The real Struldbruggs experience not an immortality of splendid youth but a never ending old age, with the usual infirmities and many more 'which arose from the dreadful prospect of never dying' (Swift 1940: 226).

When they reach the age of 80, the Struldbruggs are considered dead in law. 'Their heirs immediately succeed to their estates, only a small pittance is reserved for their support; and, the poor ones are maintained at the public charge'. Swift did not finish *Gulliver's Travels* until he was nearly 60, and it is reasonable to conclude that in this part of the book he is coming to terms for himself with the prospects of old age and death. His observation (thinly disguised as that of a Luggnaggian who had visited Japan) was that long life was 'the universal desire and wish of mankind. That, whoever had one foot in the grave, was sure to hold back the other as strongly as he could. That the oldest still had hopes of living one day longer and looked on death as the greatest evil' (Swift 1940: 225).

Swift holds up to himself and so to his readers the absurdity of human beings' fear of death and desire for long life, by spelling out for us what the prolongation of old age would be like with no prospect of death. His words strike chillingly near the bone as a description of the reality of extreme old age in the west at the start of the twenty-first century.

A historical perspective

A key theme of this book will be that the experience of housing in later life in Britain at the start of the twenty-first century is not some inevitable consequence of the ageing process but is socially constructed. To explore this idea it seems helpful in this introduction to see how economic, political, ideological and social factors have in the twentieth century affected housing issues for older people. A historical analysis shows that in the past, as now, older people's welfare outcomes were very much affected by their housing careers which in turn were affected by land prices and policies, tax policies and labour costs, dictating how much was built and at what price. A historical analysis also shows that although much has changed in the past 100 years there are important continuities.

The beginning of the twentieth century

At the turn of the century for people of all classes, rental from a private landlord was the normal form of tenure but its impact was very different, depending on class and wealth. Around 30 per cent of the population belonged to what was described then as 'the servant-keeping class'. Whether their home was an inconvenient mansion or a comfortable suburban villa, there was no anxiety about managing the home as they became older and less fit. Even when there was no family, care and support were provided by the servants or more commonly servant, normally a female, aged 25 on average (Sanders 1903: Table xxiv).

For working-class older people, the majority, the picture was less rosy. The condition of poor people's homes, whether in town or country, was generally atrocious (Booth 1894; Rowntree 1902; Crotch 1908). Inadequate water supplies and lack of sanitation took their toll of lives in summer; cold, damp, pollution and lack of ventilation in winter. Overcrowding was universal. Even worse, the lack of an assured income while having to pay for rent and subsistence caused physical and mental suffering. Just under 5 per cent of older people were resident in the workhouses in 1901, but many more dreaded the possibility. There were some occupational pensions; some rent-free housing in the country; some almshouse places with provision for subsistence and a variety of savings and insurance schemes, but none of these was adequate to provide for the majority of older people. Out-relief (payment in cash under the Poor Law) was widely given but was never enough to house and sustain an older person; it was sufficient only to augment their other meagre means. People took in a lodger, took menial poorly paid jobs, lived on their savings till these were exhausted, and did whatever else they could to sustain their homes. Financial help from families was extremely important (Thane 1998). Daughters also contributed generously. The 1 million young women in domestic service in 1901 were often supporting two sets of older people with their hard labour: their employers and their parents.

Practical help in the home for older people also came mainly from the family, and this was easier because of the nature of households. It was not that people lived in enormous extended families as is often commonly supposed. The average household size was only 4.6; this often included a lodger in poor households and a servant in richer ones. The crucial difference was that almost no older person lived alone but this did not mean that they went to live with children. The majority of older people, then as now, lived in a property where they or their spouse were 'head of household'. But when one partner died, the men often married again, frequently someone considerably younger. In other cases a son, daughter, grandchild or other relative lived with their parent and helped pay the rent.

Housing conditions for the majority of older people in 1901 were generally bad for the following reasons. The ownership of land was in private hands; enclosure, industrialization and a free market economy had created slums in town and country alike. There was a shortage of decent, affordable housing for working people because it was not a viable proposition for anyone to supply it. The rating system acted as a powerful disincentive to potential landlords. Local rates were the principal form of taxation, producing nearly double the revenue from income tax. These rates were based on the value of property, and any improvement to the property meant an increase in the rateable value.

Octavia Hill, who was widely regarded as a housing reformer because of her work in raising management standards, promoted '5 per cent philanthropy', the idea that people could invest in housing for the poor and still receive a 5 per cent return. She opposed vigorously and effectively the state provision of housing (Hill 1998: 95). However, Hill achieved investment more by force of personality than by the strength of her economic argument and was, of necessity, unrelenting in enforcement of rent payment. (Prince Albert is quoted as saying that 'unless we can get 7–8 per cent we shall not induce builders to invest their capital in such homes': Merrett 1979: 17.) Also, the number of homes provided through Hill's methods was minute compared to the need. Finally, housing conditions were bad for older people due to their inability to service rent levels. They were penalized by the poor wages they earned throughout their lives and by the failure through incompetence or downright dishonesty of many private insurance and pension schemes.

The emergence of state provision

These were the economic and fiscal factors affecting housing circumstances but there were ideological ones too. A struggle was underway between, on the one side, Charles Booth and all those who supported the idea of old age pensions, and on the other Octavia Hill, Charles Loch and the Charity Organization Society (COS), who feared that state provision would create dependency. Such debates about the relative responsibility of individuals, families and the state were very much alive at the end of the twentieth century.

The COS was founded in 1869 with the aim of coordinating charitable agencies in London to prevent the indiscriminate giving of charity and reneging by families of their responsibilities to their dependent members. The COS campaigned for the abolition of all 'outdoor relief' and a strict enforcement of the Poor Law Amendment Act. Loch (1911: 885) referred to old age pensions as 'a huge charity started on the credit of the state'.

However, despite the best efforts of members of the COS, the arguments of Booth and his compatriots won out. Although there is a popular image of Victorians as being champions of market forces, in fact they were becoming persuaded of the need to recompense for a long life of low or subsistence wages. The foundations of the welfare state were laid down at the end of the nineteenth century. Painstaking research led Charles Booth and others to believe in the value of unstigmatizing universal benefits on which older people could rely, and which would encourage family and friends to contribute what help they could, knowing they would not have to bear the whole burden. The 'independence' that this state help permitted to old people was a home of their own for as long as they live and freedom from *absolute* dependence *on their relatives*.

The postwar period

By the mid-twentieth century, older people's ability to pay for their housing had been transformed by the introduction of state-organized benefits. Old age

Table 1.1 Population changes and percentages of older people in the UK, 1901–97

	1901	*1951*	*1991*	*1997*
UK population	38,237,000	50,225,000	57,808,000	59,009,000
People aged 60+	2,876,000	7,923,000	11,988,000	12,052,000
Over 60s as percentage of total population	7.5	15.8	20.7	20.4

Source: Office for National Statistics 1999c

pensions in limited form were finally introduced in 1909, national insurance in 1911, widows' pensions in 1925; and in 1948, the welfare state introduced by the Labour government augmented pensions with national assistance. Also, the state had at last began to subsidize the building of council housing: 1.5 million council homes were built with state subsidies between 1919 and 1939 (Burnett 1986: 249). Between 1945 and 1961 councils completed a total of nearly 3 million homes – 1 million more than were built in the private sector (Malpass and Murie 1999: 55). Some of this housing was specifically designated for older people, and from 1948 onwards sheltered housing was also built (Butler *et al.* 1983).

These social changes were the result of economic and political upheaval, two world wars and very hard work by those who wanted a more just society. There were also demographic changes. Table 1.1 shows that between 1901 and 1951, the proportion of people over 60 in the population rose from 7.5 to 15.8 per cent, an increase much more dramatic than that which has occurred since 1951 but absorbed with less panic. In 1951 there was a great shortage of labour and older people, who had contributed much to the war effort, were asked to stay on in the workforce, so there was not so much discussion of the burden of an ageing population.

Despite the advent of the welfare state, older people were given lower priority than families. The amount of housing built by local authorities for older people was not in proportion to the scale of their need (Butler *et al.* 1983). Workhouses were abolished in theory, but money was not put into the 'homelike' establishments that were supposed to replace them, so conditions for those in residential care remained abysmal (Townsend 1962). Also family sizes were getting smaller and there were more older people, both single and couples, who had no younger person living with them to help. This affected all classes (the number of households with resident servants was down to 1.2 per cent in 1951: Burnett 1986: 280) but the response of the state in terms of providing home help throughout the second half of the twentieth century never approached the level of need. What is more, the seeds of the present housing circumstances of many people who are old now were sown in the 1950s and 1960s when they were young. Women were paid less than men, and had great difficulty getting mortgages, while single people of either gender and childless couples were also low priority for council housing allocation. These factors drove such households into the private rented sector, whence they could never escape. This is why so many very old people, especially women, are living today in poor condition privately rented properties. Owner occupation, the preferred tenure of the late twentieth century, is today similarly out of reach for a significant minority of older people.

Continuity and change

We need now to summarize what has changed and what has not throughout the century. Some factors of housing in later life have remained very constant. The great majority of older people have always lived as heads of households or spouses of heads of households in ordinary housing, and have been largely independent. They have consistently received more practical help from their family than from the state but at no point have the majority been living in large family groups. The numbers living in specialized housing or residential care have been consistently tiny. People without family have always been more likely to spend the last years of their lives as residents of institutions, whether workhouse, long-stay hospital, residential or nursing home. At least since the 1950s, the amount of domiciliary services to enable people to live independently has always been inadequate for the scale of need.

The major and most significant change is that in household composition. Table 1.2 shows the growth in numbers of older people living alone, from 6 per cent in 1891 to 42 per cent in 1994. Tenure change has also been striking. The number of older owner-occupiers has sharply increased. Some other changes have occurred which have greatly improved the housing circumstances of older people. The introduction of the old age pension was vital. The non-means-tested attendance allowance plays an additional crucial role at the end of the twentieth century. The slum clearance and the new house-building programmes of the 1930s, 1950s and 1970s and the provision of grants for repair and adaptation were also vital.

However, this historical perspective has to close on a fairly negative note. Towards the close of the twentieth century there was a sustained assault on the welfare state. The good effects of the social reforms described have been diluted by cutbacks in government spending, and the illusion that the housing needs of poorly paid people can be met by private finance. Equally disturbing has been the resurrection of the ideas of the Charity Organization Society about the effects of giving help, carried forward knowingly or unknowingly in government policies.

Table 1.2   Changes in living arrangements of older people, 1891–1994 (household types as percentage of all households containing at least one person over 60)

Household size	1891	1994
One person	6	42
Two persons	18	45
Three or more persons	76	13

Sources: 1891 Census; Leather
Note: Figures for 1891 based on analysis of households in Pinner, Middlesex, as recorded in the 1891 Census returns

The current policy landscape

The chapter draws to a close with a look at the curent policy landscape. Here it is possible to be more positive than the preceding historical analysis could be about housing and social welfare policies towards the end of the twentieth century. At the point when this book was being written, there was no respite from the spate of policy initiatives and pronouncements about old age which have been a feature of the social policy landscape during the 1990s and early years of the new century. Politicians continued to worry about demographic 'pressures' but the language was less intemperate than in the 1980s with its talk of 'rising tides' and 'demographic time bombs'. For example, the Labour government, when it came to power in May 1997, established an inter-ministerial group on older people as part of its project to promote 'joined up government'. In December 1997, it launched its *Better Government for Older People* initiative which aimed to involve older people themselves in inter-agency strategies and (as we show later in the book) *prevention* became a key theme in public statements with an implicit acknowledgement that there had been undue emphasis on ever increasing targeting of those in the most need. In the early part of March 1999 *With Respect to Old Age* (the report of the Royal Commission (1999) appointed by the government to examine the funding of long-term care) was published. This was a very significant event, not so much in what it recommended, but in its success in bringing together an enormous wealth of data and comment on ageing in Britain. *With Respect to Old Age* (Royal Commission 1999) has succeeded in getting the issues of old age well aired, it has focused on housing-based alternatives to residential care and it has turned its back on the notion of old people being a problem. There has also been pressure on government from other sources. Age Concern has orchestrated an influential millennium debate and Help the Aged (Harding 1997) has attempted to get older people on to the government's social welfare agenda. The latter, with its focus on social exclusion and welfare to work, appeared largely to ignore them.

The beginning of the new century thus seems a more positive period in terms of how older people are perceived than that immediately following the community care changes of the early 1990s. However, we shall be arguing in this book that, although the language may have changed, the reality, on the whole, has not. Octavia Hill and the Charity Organization Society have cast a long shadow. There is little evidence that the lessons of history have been learnt and the rationale for policies of universal provision rediscovered. The agenda of other 'bits' of government do not coexist comfortably with social welfare policies about involving older people in service delivery and placing more emphasis on prevention. Although, as this book was going to press, public spending plans were becoming more generous, housing in the public sector continues to be badly affected by the processes of residualization and expenditure on social security and social services continues to be under severe pressure. Paternalism, control and failure to listen to what older people want themselves continues.

PART I

Reviewing the issues

2

Theories, assumptions
and policies

This chapter sets out to persuade that theorizing housing, home and later life will lead to a better understanding of both the policy decisions of governments and the decisions that older people take in relation to their home environments. In Chapter 1, we have suggested that housing policy, relating to older people, is both narrowly construed and ageist; that housing and home are distinct concepts and that there are distinctive characteristics of later life which have implications for social and housing policies, although later life itself is very differently experienced. The purpose of this chapter is to develop these themes further and to provide a conceptual framework for the rest of the book.

In the mid-1980s, one of us (Means 1987) called for an expanded view of housing and home in later life beyond narrow policy concerns. Here in this chapter we continue with this challenge and review different paradigms of old age and discuss their relevance to housing studies. We argue that employing concepts from social gerontology will broaden and enrich the study of housing and later life. But we also argue that the process should be two way. Social gerontology can inform housing studies but, equally, the incorporation of a housing and home perspective into ageing studies will address a current neglect. The chapter then examines the literature on the meaning of home in later life which, in the main, has been approached from a housing perspective rather than from ageing studies. It is suggested that a more explicitly 'gerontological' approach might develop our understanding of how home is experienced. The final section of the chapter turns to housing policy and practice as it relates to older people. The policy literature, it is asserted, gives the appearance of being atheoretical; it has an aura of being value free and true. A closer examination, however, reveals that it is not without implicit theory. Despite espousal of independent living principles and an increasing critique of 'special needs', policies and practice continue to be predicated on a negative view of old age.

Different theoretical perspectives on old age

What follows is a very brief, arguably idiosyncratic and highly selective account of the more dominant paradigms of old age. The boundaries between the terms used to describe different models are not rigid. The models, as presented here, 'leak' into each other.

Old age as a problem for individuals

There are a wide range of different and sometimes competing theories of old age which focus on the individual ageing process. They derive their intellectual base from different disciplines such as biology, various branches of psychology and social psychology. Although very different, what they have in common is the assumption that old age is a problem for individuals.

The now well-accepted idea that old age, like gender and disability, is socially constructed does not have a long history. Until the 1960s, overarching theories were biological, developmental and generally located within the individual. As Lynott and Lynott (1996) have argued in a paper on the history of theoretical developments in gerontology, the 'facts' of old age some 30 years earlier were ill health, retirement, poverty or social isolation. These had to be adjusted to; they were natural phenomena. Researchers like Havinghurst (1954) developed concepts around the individual such as 'adjustment', 'activity' and 'life satisfaction'. In a roughly similar tradition, the structural functionalists posited disengagement theory (Cumming and Henry 1961). Although the work of scholars like Havinghurst (1954), Neugarten and Hagestad (1976) and Cumming and Henry (1961) can be located within sociological theory, nevertheless the social aspects of old age are underplayed. The focus is the individual older person adjusting to the problems of later life. Disengagement theory relates the changing needs of the individual to those of the social system. Central to the theory is the idea of equilibrium: 'The equilibrium which existed in middle life between the individual and his society has given way to a new equilibrium characterised by a greater distance and an altered type of relationship' (Cumming and Henry 1961: 14).

Although out of favour with many social scientists, disengagement theory lives on in everyday discourse about old age. Of intuitive attractiveness to the 'not old' is the idea of self-preoccupation or self-absorption that disengagement theorists would argue comes with old age. There must be many middle-aged individuals who have rationalized their very elderly parents' lack of participation in their younger relatives' lives in terms of remarks such as 'She is simply turning in on herself, concentrating on survival'. Similarly, in social policy and practice, debates about older people are negative, concerned implicitly with disengagement and decline. Despite the concern of many commentators to be politically correct and refer to the objects of their study as older people, the label 'the elderly' is still common currency. Policy interventions, it can be seen throughout this book, continue to be evaluated in terms of how successful they are at arresting inevitable physical and mental deterioration.

A political economy of old age

From the mid-1970s, western democracies were experiencing, to varying degrees, financial crisis in terms of rising unemployment and inflation. Significant cutbacks were made in the funding of pensions and welfare and older people tended to be seen as a burden, creating huge pressures on public expenditure (Phillipson and Walker 1986).

It was against this background that the political economy perspective of old age began to emerge. It directly set out to challenge the biomedical model of ageing with its implicit tendency to pathologize old age. At the heart of the political economy approach is the concept of the social construction of old age; the many experiences faced by older people are the product of economic and social structures such as compulsory retirement, pension policies and social and health care systems. The model is not, of course, denying biological processes; rather it is highlighting issues of power and ageism which characterize societal approaches to old age. Alan Walker (1981) coined the phrase 'the social creation of dependency' and, in similar vein, Peter Townsend (1981) developed the notion of 'structured dependency'. In the United States, Carroll Estes (1979) used the expression the 'ageing enterprise' to describe how older people are treated as a commodity, and called attention to the universal tendency to adopt age-segregated policies. The political economy perspective was immensely valuable in showing that old age is differentially experienced through class, gender and, more latterly, ethnicity. It has also challenged the moral panic in evidence in the 1980s and early 1990s about perceived sharp increases in the elderly population. Estes commented that blaming older people was seen as a means of obscuring 'the origins of problems [which stem] from the capitalist economic system and the subsequent political choices that are made' (Estes 1986: 123).

In the UK, Peter Townsend illustrated his own structured dependency thesis through his analysis of social policies for older people. He saw social and health care as a clear example of how the state imposes dependency upon older people and he saw enforced retirement as legitimizing low income and leading to socially manufactured dependency:

> The failure to shift the balance of health and welfare policy towards community care has also to be explained in relation to the function of institutions to regulate and confirm inequality in society, and indeed to regulate deviation from the central social values of self help, domestic independence, personal thrift, willingness to work, productive effort and family care. Institutions serve subtle functions in reflecting the positive structural and cultural changes taking place in society.
>
> (Townsend 1981: 22)

A key element within the political economy paradigm is the notion of ageism. For Townsend, residential care was an extreme example of institutionalized ageism but he was also critical of the dependency effects created by care professionals working in the community. Institutionalized ageism discriminates against people on the basis of their chronological age; it marginalizes older people and makes it hard for them to participate fully in society. It is not difficult to find contemporary examples of institutionalized ageism within social and housing policy. Locally delivered social care services are organized into 'Services for people with physical disabilities', 'Elderly people services', and so on. Whether a person falls into the former or the latter depends on the whether they are over or under pensionable age. Until very recently older people were discriminated against in terms of 'direct payment' policies and, despite *Better Government for Older People* initiatives, citizens' charters and the Department of Health's policies on user-led assessments, power relationships between care providers and older people are asymmetrical. In Chapter 3, a number of housing examples will be proffered of discrimination against older people.

The ageism that results from older people's structured dependency is challenged within the political economy paradigm. Older people's social exclusion can be countered by extending social citizenship principles (Marshall 1992) to older people (Leonard 1982; Midwinter 1992).

Critical gerontology

The political economy perspective on old age has received some criticism not only for being overly concerned with dependency brought on by economic disadvantage but also for its implicit determinism which sees older people as passive, even insentient, beings. Since the late 1980s the model has relaunched itself as a key component to an all-encompassing project known as critical gerontology, espoused first of all in the United States by academics like Achenbaum (1978); Moody (1988) and Minkler (1996) and in the UK by Phillipson and Walker (1987). Critical gerontology is still concerned with structural inequalities but it goes beyond old style structured dependency by proposing that the study of old age should include interest in moral concepts and in the broader issues of meaning and purpose in old age. Debates within social gerontology mirror wider discussion in critical social policy concerning a commitment not only to understand but also to challenge.

It is a position which is quite different from that of the stereotypical value free social scientist which still characterizes some social policy/housing policy research. Moody, one of the earliest proponents of the new critical approach to gerontology, sounds almost evangelical in the following:

> A critical gerontology must also offer a positive idea of human development: that is ageing as movement towards freedom beyond domination (autonomy, wisdom, transcendence). Without this emancipatory discourse (i.e. an expanded image of ageing) we have no means to orient ourselves in struggling against current forms of domination.
>
> (Moody 1988: 32–3)

Phillipson (1998) identifies three separate epistemological strands within critical gerontology which can be united through the single idea of empowerment. First, there is the political economy approach with its focus on the structural barriers and constraints faced by older people. Second, there is the humanistic or phenomenological perspective which, as the quotation from Moody (1988) implies, sees ageing studies as going beyond the scientific to include moral, ethical and existential themes. The humanistic perspective allows the employment of the concept of reflexivity (Giddens 1991): the way in which individuals both influence the world around them and modify their behaviour in response to information from the world. It looks at the meanings that older people ascribe to events and circumstances. It does not, as earlier theories had done, deny human agency. The humanistic perspective with its emphasis on subjectivity leads to qualitative or interpretative research methodologies. Jaber Gubrium's (1986, 1993) work is exemplary of an approach that privileges how very frail old people describe both the process of ageing and their present circumstances.

Phillipson (1998) labels the third strand within critical gerontology biographical. It employs the concept of the life course but can do so in different ways. Johnson (1976), for example, was one of the first to use the idea of the biographical career in which the self is made up of the different strands making up a person's life. Others, for example Ruth and Kenyon (1996), use the idea of the 'storied self' in which the individual can subject the account of their life to numerous revisions. What, however, is the common theme within the biographical perspective is the idea that people's histories – their biographies – can contribute towards understanding both individual and shared aspects of ageing over a life. Biographical data help to understand the possibilities and limits set by the historical period in which people live.

The attraction of critical gerontology is that it appears to acknowledge the importance of social and economic processes in marginalizing older people but, at the same time, to listen to and understand how individuals cope with, counteract or respond to these wider societal processes. The concept of empowerment brings together the different strands within critical gerontology; it can potentially be realized through social and economic polices concerned with redistributions of wealth and power and/or through the reawakened feelings of self-worth that ageing individuals may achieve through telling their stories.

The declining body

Developments within critical gerontology have been driven by the proponents of the political economy model who wished to address the limitations of their approach. We need to give separate consideration to approaches to old age that derive from ideas within the sociology of the body. As Oberg (1996) has noted, the body has been surprisingly absent from discourses on old age given 'not old' people's *and* older people's fears and prejudices about failing bodies and minds. Nevertheless, there is a growing literature, some of it explicitly 'postmodernist' and some rooted in earlier symbolic interactionist theories, which, at first glance, seems to be returning to the interests of the functionalists in the 1950s, namely the management of self. However, the new literature is quite different, based as it is on social, rather than psychological, theory about identity (Nettleton and Watson 1998).

From within the sociology of the body comes a different approach to the notion of ageism from that developed within structural theories of old age. It is one which is more 'experiential'. Ageism is defined by those working within the political economy perspective in terms of discriminatory social and economic polices. Some writers' approach to ageism owes more to ideas from the sociology of the body than to politico-social theory (for example Bytheway 1995). For the purposes of the aims of this book: to understand both the policy decisions of governments and the housing decisions of older people both manifestations of the word ageism are of value. In this section of the chapter we focus a little more on the experiential version.

The visibility of the 'broken down' body induces fear and denigration in people, whether they are care workers, relatives or the very old people themselves. It leads to an ageist approach, whether in research, in policy or in service delivery. For example resource allocation in social policy focuses on 'competence' as measured by Activity of Daily Living (ADL) scales and considerable emphasis is placed on the idea of 'protection'. In social research on later life, ageism is rife even among those who in their writings condemn discriminatory ageist practices. Fieldwork with frail old people is viewed as a problematic exercise. 'Youthful' researchers (Jerrome 1992) often avoid employing in-depth interviewing techniques because they are awkward about meeting old age head on (Oldman and Quilgars 1999). Challis and Bartlett (1987) in their study of nursing homes found it difficult to 'get beyond an overwhelming undercurrent of sadness' and Bytheway (1995) noted that questions are asked which confirm the researchers' own fears and prejudices about old age. Similarly, Minkler (1996) has argued, citing the American sociologist Jon Mckinlay, that researchers suffer from a malady known as 'terminal hardening of the categories'. They get the kinds of answers they can cope with because they ask the kinds of questions that fit their view of old age.

Old age can be frightening for those who are in it or for those who can see it coming. Deep old age (Featherstone and Hepworth 1989) is particularly feared because of its association with the loss of bodily controls and with Alzheimer's and other mental health problems. Featherstone and Hepworth have written extensively about the self becoming a prisoner in the ageing body which is no longer able to maintain its true identity. The tension between the inner subjective experience and physical appearance is described by the mask of ageing. The mask is pathological and the self is normal.

Old age in a postmodern society

Matters postmodern have already been touched upon in the chapter but here a postmodern perspective on old age is examined in a little more detail. We live in a postmodern time or, as Giddens (1991) would prefer it, in late modernity. It is difficult to deny that the fundamental changes that have affected western democracies since the late 1970s have implications for growing older at the beginning of the twenty-first century. The postwar welfare settlement has collapsed (Williams *et al.* 1999); globalization has brought in, among other things, new forms of economic production and within 30 years of the new century the proportion of those over pensionable age is projected to constitute one-third of the population as opposed to one-fifth at the present time (Falkingham 1997). Most relevant to this current discussion of old age and the postmodern society are the quite enormous changes which have taken place within social policy. The giants of the welfare state – housing provision, pension provision and social and health care services – which all, for a limited period after the Second World War, provided older people with some certainties and some security have been subject to a process of destabilization. Moreover, recent periods of unemployment and major economic restructuring have resulted in large numbers of people, predominantly male, leaving the workforce before pensionable age. Housing has been in the vanguard of the restructuring that has affected the welfare state. Other chapters of this book discuss more fully the impact of residualization of social housing on older people (Burrows 1999); here it is sufficient to say that council housing now accommodates disproportionate numbers of older people whose opportunities to move within the sector to accommodation which is safer and more convenient are compromised by the reduction in the supply of more attractive properties although, with specialist housing for older people excluded from 'right to buy' programmes, arguably less so than other groups. From the 1980s council tenants were encouraged via various discounts to buy their properties. These initiatives were known as 'right to buy'.

Health and social care have been subject to privatization and marketization. Continuing health care, through a process of stealth largely undebated in the early years, has been redefined as social care (Oldman 1991a) and significant numbers of older people have no choice but to trade their housing equity for places in the much expanded private nursing and residential home sector.

To sum up, thus far, being old in the postmodern world seems bleak. Old age itself has become a major source of risk and the intergenerational contract of yesteryear heavily under attack. However, a more positive view of postmodern old age can be advanced. Older people, despite income inequalities within the 55–100 age span, are better off – more likely to have occupational pensions and be owner-occupiers – than previous generations (Hancock 1997) and can, subsequently, be active players in the consumption culture which is the hallmark of the postmodern society. Gilleard (1996) notes:

> more and more older people are joining in this shopping trip searching for reasonably priced identities and personal self care plan to follow through the dangerous territory of infinite desire. Modernity had structured the identities of old people, exchanging their role in the productive processes for a guaranteed but limited security in old age. Late or postmodernity, whilst dislocating and diffusing these earlier collective social identities offers *older people the opportunity to engage more comprehensively with the project of identity.*
>
> (Gilleard 1996: 495, added emphasis)

Lifestyle, choices and identity are the key concepts of postmodernity and writers have commented that they all have relevance to older people. Featherstone and Hepworth (1989) talk about the modernization of ageing which for them means people distancing themselves from the period of deep old age. They describe a new youthful identity in old age created through renegotiating and prolonging middle age. Anti-wrinkle cream, the University of the Third Age and private retirement housing could all form part of a 'successful ageing' programme.

The positive and negatives of old age and postmodernity have been briefly set out above. The negatives, however, seem to win out. First, although there is evidence of rising affluence, it seems there is only a middle-class minority for whom choice is not a hollow concept. As Gail Wilson (1997) has wryly commented, anti-wrinkle cream consumes a significant element of the weekly state pension. Second, although the new social movements comprised of active welfare subjects are powerful mechanisms for creating strong self-identities (Williams *et al.* 1999) there is no evidence, in the UK at least, of strong 'agers' movements. Third, fundamental to postmodern theories is risk (Beck 1992); older people have been cast loose from the certainties created by full employment and relatively well-funded welfare institutions. For many, privatization of welfare institutions is not a liberalizing force but, rather, restricts choice further. Phillipson (1998: 135) has commented: 'maintaining identity is in any event a struggle for people who by virtue of illness or their residential location, may be denied the support and interaction essential to reaffirming a sense of self and identity' and 'Older people have moved into a new zone of interdeterminancy, marginal to work and welfare' (Phillipson 1998: 138).

Old age and disability

This account of the main traditions within ageing studies concludes by looking outside the discipline itself to disability studies (social gerontology's own development has been influenced by developments within both disability studies and feminist studies).

Disability studies has itself come in for criticism over the years for being narrowly focused on disability in younger life and even there on physical disability rather than on other disabilities. There are, however, very strong arguments for employing its concepts to the study of later life. Central to disability studies is the social model of disability. This is a powerful construct which can usefully be employed to challenge older people's structured dependency. Social policy and practice as it relates to older people is so often predicated upon a medical model of disability focusing on the functional limitations. By contrast, the social model of disability draws a distinction between impairment and disability. The social model does not see the 'problem' as lying within the impairment of the individual but within society itself. It is not the individual who is unable to participate in society but society which disables the individual from that participation. This message is never so compelling as in the case of housing. The house – its steps and stairs, its too narrow doors, its overall standardized design, its lack of space and so on – creates the disability. This is a very different approach from the medical model, which has a tendency to see disability as a personal tragedy and the disabled person as victim (see for example Oliver 1990; C. Barnes *et al.* 1999).

The social model of disability might be a more effective concept than the rather weak notion of citizenship (Marshall 1992) which, as a number of writers (for example Higgs 1995; Bernard and Phillips 2000) have noted, is devoid of any real political effectiveness in the context of welfare restructuring. The term 'citizen' tends to be hijacked by governments and used to justify personal responsibility for health and social welfare (Bernard and Phillips 2000). There may, nevertheless, be some objections to taking the social model of disability and applying it to the study of later life. First, disability is not the common experience of later life. Illness and disability affect a minority of older people. Second, Means and Smith (1998a) have argued that older people experience disability at the end of a 'normal life'; they thus may believe that their impairments and ill health do make a difference. However, all three of us in our research with older people have met *some* older people who deny and 'normalize' their disability.

Perhaps surprisingly, there has yet to happen a sustained debate between academics working within ageing studies and academics working in disability studies. It has simply been noted at various conferences and gatherings that there are arguments for and against a merger of concepts. Our view here, however, is that recognizing that being old is different from being disabled does not invalidate the use of the social model of disability to challenge current orthodoxy about old age. We hold this view because the social model of disability itself has moved on from its exclusively structuralist formulation and become more useful. Both disabled writers (for example Morris 1991) and non-disabled writers (Parker 1993; Oldman and Beresford 2000) have noted that issues of pain, illness and impairment should not be denied; to do so is unhelpful. We also support the social model of disability because of its affinity with the precepts of critical gerontology: that the task of the researcher is not just to understand but also to challenge.

A further concept within disability studies which can usefully be carried across to ageing studies is that of emancipatory research. Disabled writers (for example Oliver 1992) have argued that positivist *and* interpretative models of research are alienating and cannot ever contribute to the understanding of the experience of being disabled. Emancipatory research often means disabled people, not non-disabled people, carrying out research. The lively debates that have been held within disabilities studies about the appropriateness of non-disabled people studying disability seem fairly unheard of in social gerontology. Although there have been some modest initiatives (for example Tozer and Thornton 1995) which have involved older people themselves, the vast bulk of research *on* older people is carried out by 'not old' people with all the consequent ageism which can creep in. This may of course change. The scholars who contributed to social gerontology's development are now growing older. Oliver's formulation of emancipatory research may not be acceptable to those involved in ageing studies. However, a modified version of the concept would go a long way towards addressing the ageism which, inevitably, is a current feature of old age research.

Home and housing: the unifying link

The intention of the above account of different perspectives on old age is not particularly to present any one as being the only or the most superior paradigm but rather to begin to suggest their different capacities for conceptualizing housing, home and later life. Although no one model is offered as the only defining framework, nevertheless this book is informed by the view, common to a number of the theories summarized here, that old age is a social construction. We also, for the reasons just noted above, ally ourselves with critical gerontology.

The task of the rest of the chapter is to explore more fully the usefulness of theory. It can be seen from the above account of the main developments within ageing studies that there have been two broad groups of concerns mirroring the way other disciplines such as feminism and disability studies have evolved. The first broad group are about the big themes of state, economy and politics and the second about 'micro' sociological issues: the life course, cultural representation of old age, self-identity and so on. Housing and home/domestic environments have been very largely absent from social gerontology's areas of interest. Yet, home and housing seem to represent the perfect unifying link between the two perspectives on old age, macro and micro. Also the incorporation of a housing perspective will enrich the different paradigms within social gerontology. If housing has been considered at all in the past it had largely been in a technical or descriptive rather than analytical sense; for example, '87, male, home-owner for 45 years'. Below in a discussion on the meaning of home in later life the idea that housing is the link between structural and individual concerns is explored further.

The meaning of home in later life

We start by reviewing the existing literature on the meaning of home in later life. A common theme is that 'home' is of greater importance to older people than to 'not old' people. Sixsmith (1990: 177) notes: 'In some ways "home focus" can be seen as a form of "spatial disengagement" in that a decreasing social life space is parallelled by a decreasing spatial range'.

The view that old age is a time of shrinking horizons has led some writers to see the meaning of home in later life in a very positive light. Reduced mobility, reduced social opportunities as result of reduced incomes and the death of friends results in a strong attachment to home. The most famous picture of home in later life is that of Townsend's description of family life in London in the 1950s:

Home was the old armchair by the hearth, the creaky bedstead, the polished lino with its faded pattern, the sideboard with its picture gallery and the lavatory with its broken latch reached though the rain. It embodied a thousand memories and held promise of a thousand contentments. It was an extension of personality.

(Townsend 1963: 38)

Many years later Harrison and Means (1990) in a study of 29 Care and Repair clients and Langan *et al.* (1996) in a study of 31 older households from different locations and tenures found a similar attachment to home. In the Langan *et al.* research several of the respondents stressed home as a place of privacy and refuge:

> Mr: It's a place of retreat really. Mrs: . . . and home's always been a place of where you want to go back to, however humble it is. Even when we go to town, we're still glad, well I am, to get back . . . It's a place of our own.
>
> (Langan *et al.* 1996: 6)

A number of writers (Townsend 1962; Willcocks *et al.* 1987; Peace 1993) compare living 'at home' with living 'in a home'. Living in a residential home, for example, represents an assault on self and on feelings of personal autonomy and control. Living in one's home self is secure and feelings of identity continually reinforced. Home is familiar; it is the locus of control: 'To leave homes which may be inconvenient . . . would be difficult to relinquish a hold on a base from which personal power can be generated and reinforced' (Wilcocks *et al.* 1987: 8).

Home confers a set of memories. Attachment to it can be particularly strong for older women; their disability can be concealed from the world and their status of home-ownership can give them a sense of control in a world that devalues them (Peace 1993).

There is a limited amount of empirical work which would appear to question whether home in later life always generates positive feelings. England *et al.* (2000) found, in a study of people who had recently moved to retirement housing, that, for some, home could resonate with negative memories and its deficiencies barely be tolerated.

Baldwin *et al.* (1993) argue that institutionalization is endemic in the lives of old, frail people in receipt of care services whether they live at home or in a home. In both settings these care receivers have little scope for independence and feelings of control. Biggs *et al.* (1993) have highlighted circumstances of elder abuse within the home. Oldman and Quilgars (1999), in a study which explicitly compared living at home with living in a home, suggest that for some people life at home is bleak and the social isolation that is experienced depersonalizes and dehumanizes: 'A fairly grim picture of community care when in fact the people you are caring for might be in the community but they're not necessarily part of it other than through TV sets and 15 minutes visits' (social services care manager, quoted in Oldman and Quilgars 1999: 373).

Despite the examples just given above, the current orthodoxy is that home in later life is experienced very positively. However, the main problem in appraising this view is that the body of work on which it rests is fairly limited. There is very much more to do to find out how older people experience home and how they have arrived at their particular housing circumstances and how class, tenure and ethnicity, for example, have mediated their housing experiences. Moreover, there are some methodological difficulties inherent in the current literature on the meaning of home in later life. Although it is not true of all, some contributors do not engage very well with older people but make assumptions. Also, the kinds of questions asked confirm the researchers' view of later life. For example, Sixsmith (1990) seems to be operating from within the disengagement paradigm, but this theoretical position is not made explicit. Similarly, Wilson (1991) criticizes Steinfeld (1981) for fitting older people's housing decisions into models developed for younger age groups and thus, in her view, ignoring the significance of neighbourhood in older people's lives.

Proposing a research agenda

Gurney and Means (1993) have given some consideration to developing a robust framework for understanding the complexity and significance of the meaning of home. An existential perspective (neither wholly sociological nor wholly psychological) is proposed. Its attraction is that it promises a way of linking macro factors relating to housing, home and later life (political, social and historical) with the micro ones (issues such as emotional security, identity and privacy). A three-tiered hierarchy for exploring the meaning of home is presented. It is based on three levels of meanings: cultural (everyday use of the word home), intermediate (for example tenure, class, experience of lending institutions and housing market conditions) and personal meanings (personal biography). Appropriate research tools are suggested for use at each level and a research agenda proposed. Four particular issues are identified as being interesting to pursue further:

- what tenure means to older people
- whether attachment to home is a function of people's age and/or length of residence
- whether attachment to home is re-created when housing moves are made
- whether the concept 'attachment to home' is less powerful than trading down to release equity.

Although Gurney and Means' (1993) conceptualizing of the meaning of home and life is based within the sociology of housing and does not, therefore, make use of ideas from ageing studies, it is a very useful framework which could be developed. It is of value in that it provides a way of synthesizing the impact of history and structural factors on people's housing *or* ageing careers at the same time as privileging the role of the individual in mediating these factors.

Clapham *et al.* (1993) have also put forward ideas about researching home in later life. Their approach is closer to the concerns of this chapter, that is that social gerontological concepts can inform an understanding of home. However, their motivation in arguing for a sustained research programme on housing, home and later life is a little different. They wish to see mainstream housing research broadening out to include interests in housing outcomes in old age. In this chapter, however, the focus is as much about getting housing into social gerontology as it is about getting social gerontology into housing.

Clapham and colleagues argue that the traditional way of looking at housing and old age via the cross-sectional study is very limiting and says little about how older people reached their current housing position. It also says little about how the different housing experiences of future cohorts of older people will impact on their housing destinations in their old age. A dynamic or longitudinal approach which uses the gerontological concept of the life course is proposed. Like Gurney and Means (1993), Clapham *et al.* (1993) argue that a way has to be found of linking both micro and macro factors relating to housing processes. Although recognizing the problems of using it, they suggest that structuration theory (Giddens 1979) is a way of linking the relationship between choice and structure. Biographical interviews allow older people's interpretation of past events to be placed centre stage and their views on the impact of policies listened to. However, sole reliance on biography can neglect the role of social, political and economic factors in constraining human agency.

Both Clapham *et al.* (1993) and Gurney and Means (1993) have provided springboards from which to research the meaning of home in later life further. There is considerably more scope for using the different paradigms of old age to understand how older people experience housing policies and processes. For example, the political economy/critical gerontology approach can make a useful contribution to the impact of unemployment, early retirement, class, gender and so on. Studies which give more prominence to agency and more qualitative or interpretative methodologies have also a big contribution to make to understanding how older people experience housing policies and processes. Postmodern themes – reflexivity, consumption, culture and choice – are powerful constructs in the context of a changing world for older people, increasing levels of housing equity, self-provisioning and prolonged retirement. Equally the process can be reversed; the different paradigms themselves can be strengthened through taking on a housing perspective.

The section concludes with a look at tenure and mobility.

Tenure

Tenure is a powerful component of people's housing biography and yet there is a very limited knowledge of how it is experienced in old age. Statistically, the relationships between tenure, income and age are well understood (Hancock 1997) but the impact of differences and inequalities has not generally been explored. There is enormous scope for research studies which combine quantitative and qualitative methodologies. The tenure that has attracted the most attention in the housing literature on older people has been home-ownership. Tenure differences between older people and 'not older people' are now diminishing as more and more people enter old age as owner-occupiers. Much of the interest has focused around specific policy concerns – 'house rich, income poor', using housing equity to pay for care and house maintenance and repair problems. What is far less researched is the *experience* of home-ownership, although recently the Age Concern Institute of Gerontology has carried out a sustained programme which points out some of the downsides of the tenure (Askham *et al.* 1999). Saunders' (1990) controversial thesis that owner-occupiers derive ontological security from their homes, an experience apparently denied to renters, deserves revisiting in the context of older people. Although discredited by many writers including Gurney and

Means (1993), others (for example Peace 1993; Dupuis and Thorns 1996) have implicitly supported Saunders' thesis by arguing that home-ownership reinforced self-identity. Gurney and Means (1993), however, reject the concept of ontological security, replacing it with emotional security, and call for work that compares the meaning of home by tenure.

Tenure, as an indicator of social difference, deserves more attention from the different social gerontological traditions. In terms of tenure's contribution to structural inequalities and life chances it deserves to be more central to the interests of those that work within a structured dependency or critical gerontology paradigm. Topics that could be explored include tenure and ethnicity, the impact of the right to buy programmes and renting in both the public and private sectors. Of interest to postmodernists could be the new consumerism directly consequent on increased levels of home-ownership among older householders or the tensions the latter face between spending released housing wealth and or transferring it to future generations.

Mobility

There is one outstanding major theme to discuss, that of housing mobility. There is a long tradition of work in this area in housing studies but less interest in mobility and residential stability in old age but we know that older people move less often than younger households (Leather 1999). Researchers have tended to infer that this residential stability signifies emotional attachment to home or the inability to cope with the stressful processes involved in moving house. The positive connotations of moving in younger life as a result, for example, of promotion have been contrasted with the negative status passage of moving to a sheltered flat in later life implying an inability to cope (Steinfeld 1981). These issues are taken up again in Chapter 5. Here it is sufficient to say that it would be useful to explore the social facts of housing mobility and stability employing gerontological concepts. For instance, in the housing boom towards the end of the 1980s older people were moving or trading down for very explicit financial motives (Oldman 1991b) and exercising some considerable spending power. Such behaviour could be placed within a postmodern paradigm with its emphasis on consumer, choice and self-identity.

We have tried to show that housing and home are quite separate concepts and that the meaning of home is differently experienced by older people. We now turn to look at how old age is viewed in housing policy and how theorizing housing policy could help understand the policy decisions that are made.

Housing policy and old age

Policy initiatives and service provision are shaped by the assumptive worlds of policy makers and service providers (Wilson 1991). The exploration below of two key themes, independent living and special needs housing within the housing policy literature, bears out this observation.

Independent living

Promoting independence is perhaps the key principle underpinning policy and practice relating to older people. Community care polices are now urged, as other chapters in this book will show, to have a housing component such as the provision of home improvement services or the delivery of adaptations. The central objective is to maintain 'independent living' as long as possible. Thus the criticism made at the start of this chapter that housing policies are predicated upon a dependency model of old age seems unjust. Housing policies would appear to be liberating older people from the structured dependency forced upon them in the past by social care policies. Housing interventions play a part in promoting independence. A well-adapted house may well make reliance on carers less necessary and in most circumstances older people will prefer to live at home than go into a home. The influential Department of the Environment (DoE) report *Living Independently: A Study of the Housing Needs of Elderly and Disabled People* (McCafferty 1994) is exemplary of housing policy's commitment to independent living.

Its aims were to provide estimates of the housing needs of elderly and disabled people, to provide a methodology for allocating resources for subsidized housing provision for elderly and disabled people and to examine how unmet housing need can be most cost effectively met. It concluded:

> the majority of elderly and disabled people have no assessed need for any form of subsidised need or housing with care provision. Of those that do, most can be enabled to remain at home with adaptations and health and social care support but some require a move to alternative accommodation. Current specialised housing provision meets all this demand and, in fact, there is evidence of over-provision of ordinary sheltered housing. There is however, some shortage in units for those with high levels of dependency and disability and extra care requirements.
>
> (McCafferty 1994: para 86)

Before the community care reforms of the early 1990s, a continuum of care principles was dominant. In this conveyer belt ideal, older people would live at home in the community in ordinary housing until a certain level of dependency was reached. They would then move to the next stage – sheltered housing – and then, as their dependency increased, to residential care and then to a nursing home and finally death in hospital. Some considerable research effort went into establishing objective resource allocation processes that would allow this model to work properly. Of course, it never did and studies continually found that there were older people living in ordinary housing who were very much more dependent than those in sheltered housing or there were people living in residential care who were less dependent than people living in the community. *Living Independently* seems to be predicated on the 'new' community care, rejecting the idea of a conveyer belt whereby people move on to more intensive forms of provision. The 'new' community care, in theory at least, is about delivering services to people in their own homes, not requiring them to move to specialist provision.

However, now we want to assert that, despite its espousal of the principles of independent living, *Living Independently* does not represent a fundamental policy shift; housing policy continues to be predicated on a negative view of old age. To the DoE – and arguably the Department of Health (DoH) – independent living is very narrowly defined. It means living at home, consuming minimum public resources and being supported by relatives. To those who develop policies and those who provide services independent living is simply the flipside of dependent living. *Living Independently* measures need in terms of functional and clinical dependency, the 'need' that older people may have to live in good quality housing and to have socially rich lives is largely ignored. Sheltered housing is seen by the study in terms of its contribution to the dependency/independence contrast, not in terms of any contribution it might make to people's social life.

We want to argue that the phrase 'independent living', in fact, is complex and problematic and means different things to different interests. In defining independent living as living in ordinary accommodation, housing policy is ignoring a range of other meanings of the phrase that older people may themselves be working with. The paradigms of old age reviewed above could be very useful in widening the concept and also in highlighting dissonance between older people's interpretation of independent living and that of providers. Lloyd (2000), in her research on older people facing death, provides a useful conceptual framework for better understanding the dependency/independency contrast. She is critical of the policy world's obsession with independence. She singles out the Royal Commission on Long Term Care for its concerns with the 'prevention' of dependency.

A polarized view of dependency and independency does not contribute to the well-being of people at the end of life. It reinforces the idea that dependency is an abyss into which each of us must avoid falling rather than an aspect of the human condition. In the context of developing a policy on health and social care for people who are frail and dependent on others, the position adopted by the Royal Commission is highly inappropriate. It suggests that to be cared for diminishes rather than promotes one's sense of well-being and places older people who are being cared for in the position of passive victims rather than active agents in constructing their own living and dying (Lloyd 2000).

In her fieldwork, Lloyd interviewed a woman who explained that she felt less dependent, not more as the received wisdom would have it, on going into residential care. Living alone at home she had been constantly reminded of her reliance on others. In a similar vein Oldman and Quilgars (1999) have argued that social care quality assurance systems are overly preoccupied with independent living and with encouraging older people to do things for themselves. They maintain that listening more to older people would show that independent living can mean different things to different people. For some it may not mean struggling to make one's own bed but, rather, the feeling of empowerment of having someone, whom you have paid, do something for you. The hotel model of care may be anathema to professionals but welcomed by the welfare consumer.

Closely linked to the concept of independent living is another very strong, as well as closely related, theme for recent housing policy: a moving away from special needs provision.

Special needs housing

A number of commentators during the 1980s and 1990s (Wheeler 1986; Clapham and Smith 1990; Clapham 1997) have implicitly, if not explicitly, applied a political economy perspective to their criticisms of the very long tradition of specialized housing provision for older people. The following serves to illustrate their arguments: 'So called "special housing" needs and problems that are identified as age related serve to mask the real reasons for housing deprivation in old age – low economic status and the impact of certain social and housing processes' (Wheeler 1986: 217).

Special needs provision for older people is discriminatory and ageist. It gets very near to blaming older people for not being able to manage stairs instead of seeing the issue as one of the failure of architects to build accommodation which everyone can access (Stewart *et al.* 1999). In order to attract any munificence older people have to be prepared to be labelled. Sheltered housing has been particularly criticized since it highlights the special nature of older people's housing need and is seen to reinforce negative stereotypes through age segregation. Similarly, Staying Put or Care and Repair schemes focus on the 'problem' of the elderly owner-occupier who is struggling to keep their house well maintained (Clapham and Smith 1990). Special needs policies are rooted in a medical rather than social model of disability.

In recent years housing policy has responded to these criticisms. *Living Independently* adopts a negative stance towards sheltered housing. Investment in sheltered housing has declined over recent years and there has been vigorous encouragement of initiatives to support older people in their own homes. We welcome this shift away from special needs but assert that, as with the espousal of independent living, it does not represent any real sea-change in attitudes to older people. Like the argument around independent living, the argument against special needs housing has been oversimplified. There are difficulties with not recognizing that as a concept it is problematic. Governments are let off the hook by the anti-special-housing-needs argument. They can use it as a smokescreen behind which to reduce investment in ordinary good quality housing which (as Chapter 4 shows) is so crucial to the health and well-being of older people. Not only has the development of sheltered housing slowed right down but also so has public investment in ordinary housing.

A simplistic condemnation of special needs can be dangerous if it leads to a neglect of the social needs of older people. Chapter 7 provides some evidence that *some* older people will opt to live in some form of collective accommodation. An anti-special-needs approach can go together with anti-communitaire principles. Borrowing concepts from ageing studies can help unravel the complexity of special needs. A more older-people-centred approach is likely to show that different older people have different views about housing, moving and their futures, and those views may differ from the views of policy makers. There will be some older people who do not see age-segregated living as discriminatory but make a conscious decision to move to such housing. In a postmodern age, increasing numbers of older people are in a position to buy themselves 'lifestyle', such as living in retirement housing. Tulle-Winton (1999) argues that choosing to move to retirement housing represents a deliberate stratagem to cope with 'the declining body', a positive way of 'resisting the ageing process'. She adopts an explicitly theoretical approach from the sociology of the body to discuss newly retired professional people's decision to use their housing equity for purposes of coping with impending old age.

Theory and housing policy

Despite its appearance to the contrary, housing policy literature is not atheoretical, as the discussion above on independent living and special needs housing has attempted to show. It looks value free but over the years has been imbued with different views of old age. The dominant of these is a physical or biological paradigm which focuses on dependency. Although there have been policy shifts such as an espousal of independent living, a move away from specialist provision and even a nod towards older people in social exclusion debates, there has been no fundamental change in the way old age is viewed. There is very little evidence of a real commitment to stop looking at old age negatively or a strong desire to listen to what older people themselves might be saying about their housing, homes and futures. Insights from social gerontology are immensely valuable in suggesting why policy changes are cosmetic and why ageism is enduring.

Conceptualizing housing policy and old age leads to an understanding that things are not always what they seem. The discussion above has shown that the concepts of independent living and special needs housing are much more problematic than policy makers would like them to be.

Conclusion

The chapter has argued that the literature of housing and old age has tended to confine itself to relatively narrow policy concerns. It has been largely a literature about 'housing and the elderly'. A broader, richer understanding of housing, home and later life is called for so that there might be less dissonance between what governments provide and what senior citizens want. Drawing on and making more explicit the concepts of social gerontology will aid that process. Current policies and programmes are underpinned by models or assumptions of old age. These need to be made explicit. The dominant view that older age is characterized by decline and dependency and that older people are helpless or passive in the face of the welfare that is served up to them, is giving way to newer theories that see older people as reflexive beings, constructing their own identities and in some cases wielding their not inconsiderable resources to gain power and recognition. 'Housing and home' needs to be more central to social gerontology. It provides a way of resolving the tension which has characterized the discipline for some considerable time, the structured dependency versus human agency problem. It links the macro with the micro. Housing embodies the key issues of policy and politics, of economics and of history. Home by contrast is intense, personal and emotional. A study of home provides, as Philippson (1998) in his own reconstruction of gerontology implies, the perfect laboratory for a micro sociology of everyday living.

3

The housing issues of old age: different perspectives

It is one of the anomalies of housing that it constitutes a very large part of the business that the electorate chooses to raise with their MPs and yet remains such a low-profile political issue nationally. In an article in a housing journal, Simon Hughes, MP for Southwark North and Bermondsey, wrote: 'For nearly 17 years, I have had unremitting requests for help in finding homes for people without them and for transfers to better homes for families with an inadequate roof over their heads' (Hughes 2000: 11). The implication of the rest of the article is that he has been able to do very little. His situation is a common one for MPs, reinforced by the fact that, administratively speaking, housing is the responsibility of local authorities, not national government. The housing issues that have received government attention are such things as negative equity, the problems of house purchase, and street homelessness in London; the former two because they are economic issues affecting the middle classes, the latter because it is an uncomfortable embarrassment which MPs cannot avoid seeing. Most housing problems are suffered in private or in concentrated areas of deprivation hidden from the view of comfortable Britain, and have ceased to constitute collectively a political issue that will win or lose elections. This is a phenomenon that has a very profound effect on the housing and housing services provided for older people. In the rest of the chapter we consider why this gulf between the needs and aspirations of people and the priorities of those who allocate resources exists, by looking at the different perspectives of different key players. The range of people who have an interest in housing in later life is immense. Besides older people themselves, there are their families and all whose livelihood comes through providing services in the home, from gardeners and service engineers to home helps and community nurses. At a broader local level, there are councillors, planners, developers, architects, home improvement agencies, landlords of all kinds, estate agents, solicitors and those who plan locally for health and social services. Finally, there are the range of people with regional, national or even transnational remits, including politicians, civil servants and voluntary organizations. It is not possible in this chapter to consider the viewpoints of all these groups so we shall focus chiefly on the contrast between the views of older people and the perspective of those who hold decisional power at national or local levels. *Caring for People* (DoH 1989) and the guidance that accompanied the NHS and Community Care Act 1990 stressed repeatedly the need for assessments that were 'needs led' (that is, starting with the wishes of the individual) not 'service led'. This chapter, by looking at the difference in the position of the 'service users' and the 'service providers', considers the implications of such a policy in the context of housing.

The prevailing paradigm in policy and practice

Decisions to treat older people as a separate group have various implications in the field of housing, some apparently beneficial, some detrimental. Single people who find themselves homeless, for example, are not entitled to any help (except advice) from social housing providers. But if they are old, they can be classified as 'vulnerable' and offered accommodation. Right to buy policies deliberately excluded specialist housing for older people, so councils have reasonable stocks, sometimes even an excess, and the number of older people who are homeless, even though it has grown in recent years, is still very small. This means that councils are able to be generous in interpreting 'vulnerable' and will normally act swiftly to house an older homeless person (Hawes 1997: 9). There have been similar benefits to older people in areas of housing grant provision and programmes for installing insulation or security devices. By contrast, there have been policies introduced to assist disabled people in their homes from which older disabled people have been carefully excluded. The Independent Living Fund was set up in 1993 with an age limit of 65. Similarly, when the Community Care Direct Payments Act was passed in 1996, there was again an age limit of 65 on those who could apply. This age limit was removed by amended regulations in February 2000 as a result of intensive lobbying, but why was the age distinction ever made? In the sphere of housing adaptations, discrimination has been even more extreme. Social services departments, who would not consider failing to provide a young disabled adult with an accessible bath or shower, have regularly agreed policies excluding people from this provision on grounds of age (see Chapter 6 for detailed examples). The reasons for these exclusions are almost entirely economic (large numbers and high demand), but they would not be accepted so easily if society had not become unquestioningly accustomed to classifying older people as a separate category. This attitude has also helped to create a housing stock which then itself becomes a social determinant and reinforces separatist thinking.

The perspective of government

It is a problem of political science to understand how there can be a perspective of 'government', when in practice governments come and go, individual ministers change even more frequently and power is in any case divided between politicians, civil servants and the judiciary. By 'government perspective' in this section we mean the likely perspective of any individual or group of individuals who have to make or recommend decisions on behalf of the nation, whether as ministers, senior civil servants, judges or senior officials of quangos (quasi-autonomous non-governmental organizations). These positions alone are likely to affect their views, and there will be considerable consistency, regardless of party affinity or post-holder. Government is committed to taking a whole view of the nation's needs and to keeping the country as a whole prosperous. They will be concerned with true expectations, as expressed in the ballot box, rather than those expressed in opinion polls. The perspective of government is likely to be long term as far as economic issues are concerned and short term for many other things. There is not much evidence of memory in government, which is largely untroubled by a sense of obligation to older people for what they have contributed in the past.

People who are part of government are reasonably well paid, and can easily be unaware of the circumstances of those who are poor. Or, perversely, they may believe that 75p will miraculously buy something useful for a pensioner in Tyneside even though it would not pay for an hour's parking in Whitehall. More significantly, they are subject to powerful forces – national, international and transnational – that may overrule other considerations when decisions are taken. These pressures make it unlikely that the housing needs of the majority of older people will be a high priority for government spending, as these older people are neither economically powerful nor sufficiently organized and coherent to influence the outcome of elections. Where older people have become organized, as in some parts of the United States and in the Netherlands, the outcomes for them have improved.

Government is concerned with the generality of provision, not the individual. It will therefore view council or housing association homes as a national asset to be used rationally, rather than as a collection of individual's homes. Government is also concerned with equity of provision nationwide and with the policing of this. Its overriding concern will ostensibly be to obtain good value for public money spent and to be able to demonstrate this. Ministers and civil servants work, perforce, primarily from statistical information, and politicians are particularly susceptible to what has been described as 'constructs of ignorance' – the process of protecting oneself from detailed information that might complicate decision making (Nocon 1989).

Finally, it is important to remember that departmental divisions are very deeply entrenched in national government. The Labour government elected to power in 1997 coined the term 'joined up thinking' in its determined campaign to break down such barriers at the local level, but has an even greater obstacle to overcome at the national level. This is because civil servants and

ministers know they will be judged on how well they have achieved departmental cost-limitation targets rather than on how they have contributed to
the well-being of the citizens, even if this would mean long-term savings
nationally. The Audit Commission points out these anomalies from time to
time but cannot necessarily bring about change.

The government view on older people's housing

At the core of the government perspective on older people is anxiety about the
potential demands of a group who are growing in number and who are seen as
net consumers of public resources (their massive contribution being so easily
overlooked). This is despite the fact (as Chapter 1 showed) that the propor-
tional growth in numbers of older people was much greater between 1901
and 1951 than it has been since, with apparently much less fuss. In this
light, the needs of older people for housing and housing services have to be
balanced with the needs of all other groups and with the need to contain
public expenditure. For political survival, policies have to appear reasonably
beneficent while being economically acceptable to the whole electorate.
Hills gives a figure that shows the 'support ratios' of numbers of working
age people to older people projected for the year 2040 in various countries
(Hills 1993: 12, Figure 6). The figure shows that in Britain this ratio will
change much less dramatically than it will, for example, in Japan, but the
point here is that the table is indicative of the way in which the issue is considered. There is nothing fixed in stone (or biology) about the age 65, which is
used as the working age cut-off point in the table, so one swift solution would
be to alter the age of retirement. If this were done, the problem would reveal
itself as one of shortage of employment in general rather than as a problem
caused by older people. Alternatively, it could be seen as caused by a shortage
of younger people, which could be solved by permitting higher levels of immi-
gration. This is not how government chooses to see it, however, and the latter
decades of the twentieth century have seen a succession of policies designed to
address the problem of older people, not the problem of shortage of jobs, or
lack of investment in housing, for example. Three illustrations are given
here of this stance as it has been revealed in the NHS and Community Care
Act 1990, in policies for council housing and in spending on housing benefit
and support services as they affect older people.

The NHS and Community Care Act 1990, which controlled and limited
access by older people to nursing or residential accommodation paid for by
the state, was rooted in the perspective of excessive growth in demand from
older people. This growth is explored in more detail in Chapter 4. In 1998,
the DoH was asked by the Royal Commission on Long Term Care to give its
perspective on how successful the Act had been. It reported that the objective
of securing 'better value for taxpayers' money by introducing a new funding
structure for social care' was the objective that had been most successfully
implemented (Royal Commission 1999, vol. 1: 6). The example in Table 3.1
gives a further illustration of the point.

From a layperson's point of view, these seem curious answers to the question, 'are older people getting better services?' Reference to Chapter 7 of this

Table 3.1 Illustration of government perspective on services to older people

In Volume 3 of the Royal Commission Report on Long Term Care, under the heading, 'An evidence-based perspective from the Department of Health', officers of the DoH set out to answer their own question, 'Are older people getting better services compared with six to ten years ago?' Their answer was as follows:

1 The number of people aged 65 and over in residential care has stabilised.

2 Spending on residential care and nursing homes has been brought under control.

3 Many older people are being assessed in order to determine the type of long term care they should receive. The once-open door into nursing homes and residential care homes from hospital using DSS funding is now closed.

4 There is evidence that care packages for older people living at home are more efficiently meeting needs, and that services are benefiting a wider range of people.

5 There is a more planned approach to the social care of older people, facilitated by the widespread development of care management procedures.

6 Area-based qualified social workers, working as care managers, are now more closely involved in the assessments and care plans of older people.

7 The views, circumstances and needs of carers are more recognised and taken into account.

Source: Royal Commission 1999, vol. 3: 25–6
Note: Numbering added

book will show that some older people would not regard the closed door of point 3 as representing an improvement and only points 4 and 7 seem to relate at all directly to service quality. Moreover, the claim in point 4 about 'services benefiting a wider range of people' itself reveals a very particular perspective, as the same authors' own figures show that the number of people receiving home care in England went down by 37,000 between 1992 and 1996, even as the total number of old people in the population increased (Royal Commission 1999, vol. 3: 34). 'Narrower but deeper' range might have been a more honest way of explaining the redeployment of resources from a large number of people with various needs to a concentrated band of those who would otherwise have been forced into residential care. These points apart, there is nothing in this answer about better services as service users would understand them.

A critical analysis of this text and of other documents and examples in other chapters of this book would show how often government servants use the word 'better' to describe services which control or reduce public expenditure. However, this tendency is not universal. The Scottish Office, in the same section of the Royal Commission report, is recorded as being 'concerned about how successful policies have been in supporting people in the community when nursing home admissions continue to rise and there has been a drop in domiciliary support' (Royal Commission 1999, vol. 3: 8). The Audit Commission (1996) has also pointed out anomalies and perverse incentives in regard to support for people living at home. Individual politicians would also no doubt query the stance represented by this submission to the Royal Commission, but the example is important. It represents an extreme but evidently powerful element in government thinking about older people's needs and how they should be met.

Council housing: a public asset which may be reallocated to solve shortage problems

As far as the direct housing of older people is concerned, the government perspective is again primarily economic. In the early 1990s, when right to buy policies combined with no new building had created a serious shortage of family homes to rent, government began forcefully to promote the concept of 'under-occupation', aimed primarily at older people still occupying their family home after their children had moved out. Local housing authorities were required to make an assessment of under-occupation and to set targets for achieving a better match between households and property size (DoE 1995). Under-occupation was defined as having two or more bedrooms surplus to needs (Mellett 1996: 4:21). Because a married couple are considered to need only one bedroom, an older couple in a three-bedroomed house who sleep apart and have one spare bedroom in which to put visiting children, grandchildren or friends are judged to be under-occupying. Tenants' incentive schemes (payments to tenants who are willing to move out of property in great demand) were introduced to encourage (though not force) people to move. The Housing Green Paper (Department of the Environment, Transport and the Regions (DETR) 2000a: 11:76) describes another under-occupation pilot scheme being tried out from April 2000 in the London boroughs of Croydon, Haringey and Newham. Under this scheme tenants on housing benefit who move to suitable cheaper housing will be entitled to a lump sum of about half of the housing benefit savings that would be expected over three years. The scheme will run for three years, and government 'will look carefully at its results to see whether giving Housing Benefit tenants a positive financial interest has a behavioural impact'.

The government perspective here is that public resources must be used efficiently and that the government of the day has a right to put pressure on secure tenants and cause a reassessment and redistribution of resources, even when these resources are people's homes. This applies only to the public sector, however.

Public spending on housing benefit and support services as they affect older people

In 1996, when the old age pension was around £70 per week, the average housing association assured rent was £50.13 and the average unfurnished market rent was £68.39 (Wilcox 1997: 150). Subsidy, either in constructing the housing, or to the person in the form of housing benefit, was clearly essential for anyone mainly dependent on the state retirement pension who needed to rent their home. During the 1990s, councils were not allowed to build and housing associations were required to increase rents and to borrow more and more of the capital they needed in the open market. This was intended to reduce government input into housing; indeed, between 1980 and 1995 the capital investment by government in housing fell from £12.1 billion to £4.9 billion. But this did little more than transfer the cost to the Department of Social Security (DSS), as the annual costs of housing benefit rose from £5.4 billion to £14.7 billion between 1986 and 1996 (Wilcox 1997: 150, 79, 187). As the Housing Green Paper (DETR 2000a) put it, in England the balance moved from 84 per cent bricks and mortar subsidy and 16 per cent personal subsidy in 1979, to 27 per cent bricks and mortar subsidy and 73 per cent personal subsidy by 1998–9 (DETR 2000a: 11:2).

The reaction of government to this trend was to look for ways of reducing the cost of housing benefit. Measures introduced through the Housing Act 1996 included restricting the amount of space for which housing benefit would be paid in any new tenancies and setting 'local reference' rents for an area, leaving tenants to find the difference out of money intended for their minimal sustenance needs. The idea was that tenants would negotiate lower rents with their landlords, or move to cheaper accommodation, regardless of its availability, or of the costs of moving. The government perspective was to reduce the cost to the public purse and the effect such measures would have on older people does not appear to have been much considered.

Despite evidence of the hardship caused by these measures, especially to people in the private rented sector, the proposals that nobody receive the full costs of their rent in housing benefit, but that they make up the difference from their other income, continue (DETR 2000a: 11:61, 11:70). One proposal seems superficially reasonable in suggesting that people could receive 80 per cent of the actual cost and up to 25 per cent of the average rent costs of the area in additional income support. But statistically, this proposal would be bound to leave many people short of enough money to pay the rent because, in the nature of averages, as many people would be above the average as below it and 5 per cent is a very small margin. People who had lived many years in a slightly nicer part of a local area could find themselves cruelly hit by such a policy, as some already have been following earlier 'reforms'. Government concern about the benefit trap for younger people, because housing association rents are so high, is fair and reasonable but people who have retired from work need policies with a slant that reflects their different position. In fact, the Green Paper does make a proposal to this effect:

> Recent announcements of organizational changes to focus services on client groups (a pensioner unit and a working age service agency), also mean that we must make sure that Housing Benefit is delivered as part of the client group approach. Our priority for Housing Benefit is to ensure that the service to customers improves as part of these other changes. One option would be to split the Housing Benefit caseload into age-related groups to integrate them into the work of the respective service delivery units. It would also give us the opportunity to adapt Housing Benefit to the specific and differing needs of the two groups. But changes of this magnitude, which would affect Housing Benefit customers, local authorities and landlords take time, planning and money, and require a focus both on the future and on maintaining and improving the current service. So whilst we welcome views to start this

debate, we would want to be persuaded that such an organizational change is, overall, beneficial.

(DETR 2000a: 11:21)

The worry here is that although the concerns about older people are flagged up in the consultation paper, changes that are driven primarily by the desire to save money tend to take place regardless of such concerns, often masked with bland hopes that the needs of vulnerable groups will be borne in mind.

The other method by which government proposed to reduce housing benefit costs at the end of the twentieth century was to exclude support services from housing benefit. This followed a ruling in the Divisional Court in 1997 that housing benefit was for 'bricks and mortar' only. A cash-limited budget will instead be allocated to social services authorities so that 'support' may be allocated to individuals on the basis of assessments, as in the general model of community care. The proposals were outlined in the policy paper *Supporting People* (DSS 1998b) and were being introduced at the beginning of the twenty-first century. Bearing in mind the 25 per cent reduction in a decade in numbers of older people receiving services in their home that followed the introduction of community care assessments, this policy does not bode well. Cash-limited rather than demand-led budgets have obvious benefits for government but are dangerous if they are accompanied by a refusal to consider the consequences, or if they are considered in the kind of way illustrated by Table 3.1.

All these attempts to reduce the cost of housing subsidies fail to accept the economic realities of housing poorer people in a society with such an uneven distribution of incomes. The lesson the Victorians took so long to learn, that the market unassisted by redistributive taxation could not meet the housing needs of those who had never been paid enough, is in danger of being forgotten again. We said earlier on that government collectively is not strong on memory. In this instance, one of the things that needs to be remembered is that through most of the twentieth century women were not paid equally for their work, so that women who are over 70 at the start of the twenty-first century have probably been underpaid all their working lives (or forced, as teachers were, to leave work if they got married).

Perspectives at local levels

Those who have decisional power at local levels, whether they be councillors or managers in housing, health or social services, are often caught between the decrees of central government, and their knowledge of the needs and views of those they are trying to serve. As central government now controls the finances for virtually all services, with such powers as capping local authority spending and the threat of personal surcharges for councillors who do not comply, the dominant influence is likely to be that of central government. It remains to be seen, however, whether devolution or initiatives to increase the influence of local people will do anything to redress the balance.

The viewpoint of housing managers

The primary tasks of senior management in any organization are to look after the assets, pursue and develop the core business of the organization and plan for the future. The starting point for senior housing managers is the stock their organization holds and existing financial obligations. As they are likely to have to meet considerable debt repayments (for money borrowed to build or refurbish the stock they already hold), their first concern must be to maximize income by letting as many properties as possible and ensuring that rents are collected. This objective is reinforced by the system of targets for rent collection and for numbers of 'voids' (unlet, empty properties) which are monitored by the DETR and the Housing Corporation respectively and are likely to affect the grant the provider receives.

The twin obligations to make best use of existing stock and maximize rental income will inevitably affect the viewpoint of senior managers about the housing needs of older people. They will want to make the best use of the stock not just for financial reasons, but in order to help as many people in housing need as possible. Directors of council housing departments, in particular, have since 1979 lost much of their best 'general needs' housing through right to buy, with no prospects of replacing it, and have been left with a disproportionate number of less popular dwellings. This is doubly hard, because there was usually a profit from the rental of popular housing in good condition which could be used to subsidize repairs to the less good homes. If, therefore, a social landlord has a number of unlet one-bedroom flats, a large number of families waiting for accommodation and a number of older couples or single people occupying the homes they had when their family was larger, it is not surprising that the landlord would want to try to persuade the older people to move. Their perspective is one of making best use of the whole stock. If tenants have secure tenancies, they cannot be forced to go, but besides the tenants' incentive schemes, other forms of pressure may be used. For example, all disabled tenants, including older people, have a right to apply for disabled facilities grant to adapt their home. But many housing authorities impose an upper limit far below the statutory limit of £20,000 and suggest to the tenants that, if it costs more, they should accept a transfer rather than adaptations.

Dealing with unpopular stock or hard-to-use buildings

Housing managers also have to find ways of using expensive mistakes from the past. One widespread solution to the unpopularity of high-rise housing for families has been to create 'vertical warden schemes': tower blocks let exclusively to people over 50 or so, with secure entry systems, a warden and sometimes a common room, laundry or other facilities. Some of these have proved popular and successful, but it is probably fair to say that the starting point from the managers' point of view was primarily the need to find a use for the blocks.

Allocation and transfer policies

All social housing providers have publicly available policies which guide their decisions on allocating any vacant property. For many years this was done in simple date order, and in a few authorities this is still the case, with councillors taking a direct interest and sometimes exercising discretion. Much more common in the 1980s and 1990s, however, has been the concept of allocating according to housing need, with points awarded for different aspects of need, such as overcrowding, lack of basic facilities or serious medical problems. The 'need' that is judged by these systems has traditionally been strictly 'housing need': that is, whether the applicant lacked sufficient bed space as defined by the allocating landlord, and/or the use of basic facilities. Absolute priority in such a system is given to those who are literally homeless, but where there is an extreme shortage of housing, this priority is restricted to those who are also vulnerable in some way, and who are judged not to have made themselves 'intentionally' homeless. Allocation policies vary over time and from place to place, depending on supply and demand, but there is rarely any room in the systems for taking social factors that might affect older people into account. Managers cannot afford, for example, to take much notice of letters from older tenants' doctors requesting transfers to ground floor accommodation on the grounds of arthritis as such instances are so common. Similarly, older people who are private tenants or owner-occupiers will be unlikely in over-subscribed authorities to secure council housing, because they already have a home. The home they have may be completely unsuitable – cold, hazardous, expensive or far too big – but most social housing landlords will not have systems for giving consideration to such factors. Nor will they be likely to help when a couple who are existing tenants of a one-bedroomed property request two bedrooms on the grounds that sharing a room has become intolerable (for example in cases where one partner has dementia). In most housing points systems, one bedroom meets a couple's housing need and that is the end of the matter.

In many authorities, on the other hand, under-occupation by older tenants attracts a considerable number of points and assists these tenants to secure a transfer. This is not applied to owners who under-occupy, however, because the high number of points are focused on the release of a council family property, not the needs of the older person as such. This illustrates the complexity and contradictions of the allocations policies that housing managers have to apply. If councils were permitted to buy the properties of owner-occupiers who wanted to become tenants, the policies could be very different. Similarly, the seaside and country homes for older tenants of London boroughs (described in Chapter 6) are allocated according to the need of the borough, not according to the merits of the older person's case. Priority goes to people living in boroughs with the highest demand for housing, and to people whose move will release a family property. A single older person who has only ever been allocated a one-bedroom flat therefore has no chance of being allocated a seaside bungalow. A policy that is ostensibly for older people is really designed primarily to meet other needs. The Housing Green Paper (DETR 2000a) proposes a liberalization of allocation policies, but at the local level the ability to change policies will continue to depend chiefly on whether there is sufficient stock to allow for choice.

Assessing future needs and planning development

When housing planners consider the housing needs of the whole population of their authority, they are able to be much more positive, creative and people focused than those who have to administer the existing stock within a tight framework of rules. Housing investment programmes and housing associations' annual reports show that there have been considerable efforts to remember the needs of older people in planning for the future. A number of councils and housing associations were ahead of the government in insisting that all new housing or a good proportion of it be built to 'Lifetime Home' standards, with level threshold, wheelchair-wide doors and a downstairs toilet even in a small house (Heywood and Smart 1996: 44).

Perspective of housing managers concerned with repair and improvement

How do housing managers or environmental health officers who are responsible for repairs in either the public or the private sector view the needs of older people? The major issue for these housing professionals, whether they deal with privately owned housing or properties they manage, is the stock rather than the people in it. The files are normally kept in terms of the address of the property rather than the name of the occupant, and renewal approaches will give priority to areas where the most stock is in poor repair rather than 'pepper-potting' (repairing scattered properties). This makes sense. Blocks of housing have to stand or fall together, and renewal of whole terraces or upgrading of whole areas are necessary if money is not to be wasted doing up individual homes in blocks which are subsequently demolished. Despite this focus on the stock, there is evidence that within all tenures officers understand that major repair work may be too disruptive for some very old people to bear, and that work should be modified in such instances. There are other differences of viewpoint, such as the question of the professionals' attitudes towards owners who do not maintain their properties, their ideas of what is important in a house and their judgement about what it is reasonable to spend on improvements.

The perspective of managers in social services and joint departments

What have managers in social services to do with older people's housing? The answer is, a very great deal. They are commonly responsible for the assessments for adaptations (and always, legally, for ensuring they are provided). They are also responsible for arranging the domiciliary services that enable older people to manage in their homes. But social services departments are driven by performance targets, massive responsibilities and budgets that bear little relation to the levels of need they are supposed to meet. They are also, in a way that does not generally apply to housing managers, involved in a risky business where mistakes may cause deaths, after which scapegoats may be sought. These factors tend to create a climate within social services departments where the correct following of procedures may be more important to managers than the outcomes for clients. These issues inevitably affect the perspective of social services managers.

The slogan 'priority to those in greatest need' , with its companion 'targeting', became common in policy documents in the 1980s and 1990s as resources were cut back. Although it sounds reasonable, in practice it is used to disguise the refusal of services to many in great need. The definition of 'greatest need' is also open to question, as it tends to be defined in terms that are of economic importance to government, rather than anything to do with the quality of life of people in need of services. It has been used increasingly to justify the refusal of services even when they are statutory rights. In regard to adaptations, this has led some social services managers to substitute their own policies for the legislation. For example, a community care charter from Derbyshire, produced jointly by the social services and health authorities (undated, but circa 1996–7) listed the eligibility criteria for receiving adaptations. Services would be provided only to cases that involved serious risks to health and safety, terminal illness, facilitation of discharge from hospital or residential care, or preventing admission to the same. At no point in the charter are the rights of the disabled person under the relevant 1989 or 1996 Housing Acts mentioned. Similar policies are found in many other authorities (as will be discussed further in Chapter 6). This example reflects the view of social services and health managers that their prime tasks as agents of both central and local government are to reduce admissions to residential or hospital care and to prevent serious accidents in cases where they might be held responsible.

As far as domiciliary services are concerned, the perspective of the managers again focuses on managing resources, but there is also some evidence of a culture or habit of refusal. For example, in the Fife users' report (Barnes and Bennett-Emslie 1997) social services managers responded to the finding that the elders consulted wanted very much a service that would clean windows and change net curtains, as these were the things they could not do themselves. One manager said, 'I would like to see them move on from windows, curtains and bulbs'. Another is quoted as saying: 'We have to constantly explain to people that to clean 10,000 windows once a month for one year would cost £2 million' (Barnes and Bennett-Emslie 1997: 43). If this sum is analysed, however, it works out at £16.66 per dwelling per month! This does not sound like an objective argument, unless window cleaners in Fife in 1996 charged three or four times the going price elsewhere. It suggests that mixed in with fair and rational points there may be a resistance from managers to user views that is not always itself wholly rational.

Other managers said they felt that the panel members were not necessarily representative of service users, and they quoted satisfaction surveys in support of their view. They also felt the panel members were giving 'opinions without responsibilities' and that they should test and rationalize their view of the need. Some of these comments are perfectly fair, but there are also

suggestions of strongly entrenched positions. Clark's evidence of the importance of clean net curtains to the older people in her study (Clark *et al.*
1998: 26) had not been produced at the time of this report, but some of
these managers displayed a resistance to listening to similar evidence from
their own service users. Of course this resistance is not universal. There
were managers in the Fife study who welcomed the report and made many
positive comments. But those who worry about power relationships between
clients and professionals in the caring service will see a too familiar pattern in
the negative responses to user requests illustrated here.

There was at the start of the twenty-first century, however, a development
which showed an authority taking a different approach entirely. Cornwall
social services department decided to drop assessment in most community
care requests and adopt instead a policy of recruiting and training special assis-
tants, giving them devolved budgets and empowering them to give people
what they asked for without any further questions or assessment. This was
after research revealed that this was what the assessment process was in
any case delivering but with a six-month delay and considerable bureaucratic
costs (Druce 2000). It will be revealing to see how many authorities follow
Cornwall's lead.

Councillor perspectives

People have traditionally become councillors to serve their local community,
to protect particular interests in that community or to start a political career
which they hope may lead to Parliament, or for a mixture of any of these
reasons. Even those who are mainly interested in local issues are likely to
have to join a political party if they are to have a chance of being elected.
Once elected, moreover, they will normally find that loyalty to the party is
expected to take priority over loyalty to the local electorate, for without
party support the councillor will have no chance of securing any long-term
influence or responsible post. They are forced to consider issues from a
council-wide perspective, to be reasonable about the needs of areas other
than their own ward and to take financial constraints and political deals
into account. On the other hand, local councillors, especially district or
borough councillors, are accessible to their voters and susceptible to criticisms
in the local press, and may, in private, be able to influence the party line on a
topic. The problem in British politics in the last decades of the twentieth
century, however, was that local parties themselves had increasingly little
freedom to manoeuvre.

In an unpublished study of joint working in housing and community care
by Heywood and Smith (commissioned by the DETR in 1998) an interview
was carried out with a group of councillors from the housing and social
services committees of a unitary authority. They came from the three main
political parties in England and spoke with almost complete unanimity in dis-
cussing the services they were able to give to older people. Their viewpoint
was that their hands were almost completely tied by central government,
and that they had neither freedom nor power to stray far from the paths
laid down for them. Spending cuts imposed not by local voters but by central

government had forced them to sell off old people's homes, privatize most of the home care services and introduce charges. No one expressed a view that any of these changes had been beneficial to the older people, but all felt they had had no option and that their main function had been to limit the damage. The frustration expressed by this group of members is reflected nationally in the high numbers of people ceasing to be councillors.

From 1999 onwards, however, starting in Wales, the system of local government has been changed ostensibly to give more power to a mayor and smaller cabinet group of councillors (exact details varying according to local preference). Whether these changes will alter the power of local authorities *vis-à-vis* national government, to build houses or provide services if they choose, remains to be seen. Without the power to decide for themselves on local taxation levels this is very unlikely. Such freedoms are more likely for those who serve in the new regional assemblies in Scotland and Wales.

Councillor perspectives on the housing issues of older people: some contrast between county councillors and district councillors

In areas where there are two tiers of local authority, the responsibility for housing as such lies with local districts while social services are provided by the wider county authority. In such cases, the district councillor is likely to be more accessible and better known than the county councillor because they serve a smaller area and normally live locally. Research into the funding of adaptations revealed how powerfully this difference could affect the housing of older people. It found that between 1990 and 1994, at a time of shrinking budgets and extreme pressure on housing departments from a government doctrinally opposed to council housing, average expenditure by local housing authorities on adaptations for their tenants rose from £13,000 to £32,000 per 1000 properties owned. The vast majority of these were for older people, and the money was found by transferring money from general repairs or planned improvements and/or by increasing rents. These decisions, according to the officers who gave the figures, were made by councillors choosing to give priority to disabled older tenants and having the power to do so within the ring-fenced and free-standing housing revenue account (Heywood and Smart 1996: 42–4).

Further research would be needed to establish the processes by which councillors in different districts around Britain reached similar decisions, and how much they were influenced by pressure from constituents, but the hypothesis that this was an example of the democratic process at work is worth considering. Social services councillors at this time should have felt under similar pressure to reduce the lengths of waiting times for assessments for adaptations (anything up to four years in some areas, and the largest single issue raised in complaints to the local government ombudsman), but the funding research did not show any examples of county councillor pressure producing enhanced expenditure for this purpose until there was a new source of funding, special transitional grant, introduced in 1993, which made action fairly easy.

The perspective of front line workers

The category of front line workers includes district nurses, housing officers, home-care staff, wardens, occupational therapists, the staff of home improvement agencies and all other people whose work regularly brings them into the homes of older people. Like councillors, front line workers are much closer to the position of older people than are senior management or those in government. The examples given here relate to only one group, the home helps/home carers, but are intended to stand as an illustration of the kinds of considerations that affect all these workers.

The perspective of front line workers is likely to include three main elements. These are first, the need to earn a living, keep the job and survive the working week, second, the desire to give a good service to older people, and third, for many, extreme frustration at the policies that prevent them from doing what is needed. The need to keep a job means that workers will mostly abide by the rules set by management, even when the rules conflict with their humane instincts or better judgement. They also know that they have to get through their case-load and balance the needs of all their allotted clients, however great the need of one may be.

Desire to give a good service keeps many people in these hands-on jobs which are so important and so under-rated. A large study of home helps carried out in 1970 showed that many home helps (as they were then) were doing extra work in their own time (Hunt 1970). The 1970 study discovered from the home helps of the time that they were frustrated at not being allowed to spend longer with clients or do the jobs the clients in general most wanted. They would also have liked to vary what they did to suit people's individual priorities. Anecdotal evidence suggests that this trend continues. The letter quoted in Box 3.1 picks up this point among others.

Box 3.1   The experience of home carers, 1999

In 1999, a letter from the relative of an older woman receiving domiciliary care from a provider agency 'purchased' by social services was published in a local paper, the *Gloucestershire Echo*. The writer said

> Carers come and go with this agency, most of whom are extremely kind and caring. The reason most people give for leaving are the awful conditions of employment and difficulties in receiving payment for work done. The hierarchy of this agency seemed to have no idea what caring meant or dignity, safety, hygiene and training. As a matter of interest, can anyone tell these poor carers how they are supposed to cook a full lunch and prepare a sandwich and salad tea with hot drinks in the 30 minutes dictated by Social Services? . . . failure to provide in this time results in carers using their own time to complete the task.

Front line staff are better placed than any group, other than older people themselves, to know what is needed, yet their views are not usually sought or heeded. In particular, they will be aware of the psychological needs that they are meeting but which are not officially part of the job. In the intervening years since Hunt's (1970) study, there have been no fundamental changes to alter the key points here, except an ever greater restriction on what may be done and worsening conditions of employment as a result of privatization.

The views of older people

The practical issues illustrated in Box 3.2 are typical of the findings of a range of reports produced by or in consultation with older people (for example Wilson *et al.* 1995; HOPe (Health and Older People Group) 2000; Oldman 2000a) and relate to topics which will be explored more fully in Chapters 5, 6 and 7. A quick glance will show how the views here expressed conflict with the national and local government perspectives that older people should move to smaller properties, not receive help with housework or gardening, not be a priority for bathing adaptations and always be assessed before being given a service. Certain themes emerge from the issues within Box 3.2. These include independence and a sense of control, home as a symbol of self, loneliness and issues of mortality and immortality.

Independence

'Independence' is the first key word, and it is interwoven with ideas of retaining 'control' and, less explicitly, status. Independence is a problematic word, as Chapter 2 tried to show. Middle-aged people do not usually need to worry about independence in their housing as they are assured of it, unless they have to face the miseries of repossession or eviction. It is a factor of importance to young people who want a home of their own, to anyone forced by lack of housing or cultural pressure to live in a relative's or friend's house and to older people because of the fear that frailty or poverty may cause them to lose it. Independence is 'being in my own home, my own space. That I've still got a bit of control over my own life – that's what's important to me'; 'I don't want to go into care, if you know what I mean. You know, going into care and being looked after and being told what to do' (Clark *et al.* 1998: 16, 17). 'At the moment I don't feel independent: don't like it at all' (Heywood *et al.* 1999: 105). 'I moved because I wanted privacy, quiet and independence' (Toffaleti 1997: 12).

As people become, with age, both less fit and less well-off, so that they are not so able either to manage the upkeep of their home themselves or to pay others to do it, the fear of becoming dependent or 'a burden' grows. Psychological studies of giving and receiving in human societies show how normal this fear is; people will go to considerable lengths to return kindnesses, favours and services that are not paid for in cash so as to be free of obligation to another person (Avila and Combs 1985). In Chapter 2, we described how differently the term 'independent living' is interpreted by the state and by older people. Clark's study reinforces this point. It shows that while some

Box 3.2   Some practical housing issues presented from the perspective of older people

'When will the authorities realise that older people need more space to move around, not less – for example for walking frames, walking sticks and wheelchairs' (Oldman 2000a: 23, quoting a council tenant aged 81). Domestic help should be seen as the crucial preventive service it undoubtedly is; a new initiative is essential to ensure that it is available to older people who need it (HOPe 2000: 11). In a Scottish study looking at reasons why older people in rural areas moved into sheltered housing, or sought to do so, the problem of maintaining a garden featured as a major factor, well ahead of a desire for warden services (Age Concern Scotland *et al.* 1997)

> the bathroom is one of the more important aspects mediating the housing satisfaction of older people . . . even at relatively low levels of disability or where there was no disability at all, it was sometimes felt that having . . . at least the toilet on the ground level . . . was a real advantage . . . With astonishing frankness, several respondents gave accounts of the difficult time which they had in doing something as simple yet as necessary as having a bath . . . Quite a few respondents complained that their bathrooms could be very cold.
>
> (Wilson *et al.* 1995: 30)

An adviser to the HOOP project (Housing Options for Older People: see Chapter 5), who was himself retired, said that the researchers and service providers needed to understand that one feature of old age affecting housing issues was unpredictability. A person might be perfectly well one day, but then be suddenly struck down by illness or accident and need a great deal of help, even if only for a fairly short time. This being the case, services needed to be flexible to be able to respond to emergencies and not to depend in all cases on assessments that took a long time to arrange. Other work has shown older people may hold on to help they don't need, or even want because they know how long it would take to get a service restored if they should have a relapse (Clark *et al.* 1998: 31).

older people set out to secure all the help they need from within their family, so as to be wholly independent of the state it was much more common for older people to want their due of help from the state so they could remain reasonably independent of family or friends. Within Britain's welfare state, older people can and do claim they have paid in advance throughout their lives in labour, national service, taxation and national insurance payments and that their independence will not be compromised if the state keeps its side of the social contract by providing some services. What people do dread is the idea of losing control over their own lives and 'being told what to do'.

In listening to the language of the older people, Clark learnt that what was often wanted was not 'care' but 'help': just enough help of the right sort to enable people to retain their precious independence (Clark *et al.* 1998: 55). The word 'help' implies that the older person remains the prime mover, remains in control and actually wants the minimum possible, covering only the things they cannot do for themselves or cannot do easily, or the times when they cannot do things. Remaining in control is a theme that is made more explicit in a report produced for Help the Aged by a group of older people: 'The whole concept of home care needs to be reviewed to ensure that it provides a properly supportive personal service *with greater control in the hands of the user*' (HOPe 2000: 11, added italics). These points are philo-sophically and practically in direct conflict with the idea of external assess-ment. To respond to them, services would need to be on demand and controlled by the person seeking help. Independence would not be a concern, of course, if old age did not bring with it the anxiety about managing a house – climbing the stairs, getting out of the bath, paying the bills, maintaining and running it generally.

> For those experiencing increased disability or ill-health, the burdens of independence and of financial pressures were exacerbated. Being increas-ingly unable to attend to matters themselves, they became more depen-dent on others and had the worry of finding reliable people to help with home maintenance or gardening.
>
> (Ashkam *et al.* 1999)

Older people have to live with the uncertainties of not knowing how long they will live, not knowing what may befall them or how costs may rise and therefore not knowing how long their money will last. These uncertain-ties make planning difficult and are exacerbated by their feelings of uncertainty of provision if they should need more help at a future date.

These are some of the key issues that lie behind the question of inde-pendence. Worry is half the problem, which is why the existence of reliable services is so important. One person, asked in the HOOP study (see Chapter 5) whether she was confident that help would be there when she needed it replied, 'Yes now I know Stay Put' (the name of her local home improvement agency). This is the kind of confidence that ought to be felt about a range of services, if the psychological needs of older people are to be met.

Home as a symbol of self

Research studies during the 1990s captured a feeling, common among older people, that their home represents themselves and the achievements of their lives (see Chapter 1). 'One of the greatest achievements in this country is to own your own property and pay for it. My property was fully paid for and it was time to put my feet up and relax. Everybody has a dream. Mine was to own my own home, fully paid for' (African Caribbean man, quoted in Heywood and Naz 1990: 104).

> The house was either symbolically, and for some actually an indication of the effort they had put into a life together with their partners. Some clients talked of the steady way they had kept the house in good repair and in some cases transformed it over the years.
>
> (Gurney and Means 1993: 124)

This identification of the home with self is a vital element in understanding the perspective of older people on housing issues. For example, if the house is a symbol of achievement, failure to care for it may (as a corollary) be seen as a sign of failure, and this is what makes the issue of housework, decorating and maintenance services so important. 'Well you go down if you let the house go down, don't you? If you're not troubled about the house, you're not troubled about yourself are you? No you must keep over the Plimsoll line, dear, keep yourself up regardless' (Clark *et al*. 1998: 19). Clark and her co-authors conclude that for the generation of women they interviewed, housework had all their lives been a skilled occupation in which they took great pride. The problem of changing net curtains was the most mentioned single housework task in their study and the consequences of being unable to do it or to get help to do it were extremely serious. 'Mrs Smith, a widow aged 81, became tearful as she explained that her curtains "were filthy"' (Clark *et al*. 1998: 26). Apart from any symbolic importance, it has been estimated that dirty net curtains may exclude up to 30 per cent of the daylight. Other research has shown that inability to keep a house clean in general is one reason given by older people for their move into sheltered accommodation (Jones 1999: 5).

If a clean house and clean curtains are important to someone, and they are forced to watch their home's decline, it will emphasize greatly to them their sense of helplessness, and the power of those who tell them it is not important. The American psychologist, Seligman, studied the high number of 'unexpected deaths' in those who were admitted to old people's homes against their will or feeling they had no choice. He concluded: 'I suggest that such deaths no longer be seen as unexpected. We should expect that when we remove the last vestige of control over the environment of an already physically weakened human being, we may kill him' (Seligman 1975: 106).

Loneliness

Loneliness is a serious problem in old age. This is perhaps worst of all for those who lose someone who shared their home – whether spouse, partner, sibling or friend. But deaths of brothers and sisters, children and friends who did not share the home but were close and special can also be terrible. In other cases serious illness or someone moving away can be as bad in their effects as death in leaving another person forlorn. Karn's research suggested that 'loss' is more of a problem than 'isolation': the proportion of widowed people who said they were sometimes or often lonely was far higher than the proportion of those who had always been single (Karn 1977: 90–2).

Those who have always lived alone as adults may be used to coping but can still suffer worse loneliness as their ability to go out or to ask people in reduces, or as loss of hearing or sight reduces their ability to be sociable. 'It's when you're older dear, you need someone to come in and help you . . . you feel as though you're on your own and it's an awful feeling' (Clark *et al.* 1998: 39).

In the HOOP study of 65 people aged 59–90 (see Chapter 5), 'having enough company' emerged as a key theme. Such a finding certainly reinforces the message that loneliness may be one of the most important housing issues of all. In this context, the ability to have family to stay becomes all the more important. With many families dispersed around the world, the ability to put up a relative who has come from Australia, Jamaica or Pakistan (or even Wigan) is of importance to many older people.

The importance of legacies

In some faiths where there is no belief in resurrection after death, it is felt that a person's immortality is maintained through the lives of their descendants. Perhaps even when this is not an explicit thought or belief it is still a sub-conscious view natural to human beings as breeding itself is to all animal creatures. Older people tell and retell family stories, wanting their children and grandchildren to remember them, to pass them on. In this way they help to preserve the memory of their own parents and grandparents as well as something of themselves. They also pass on precious things that 'belonged to my mother' or 'came from your great-grandfather' and such gifts are usually treasured by their recipients, because of the provenance even when they are not worth a lot in financial terms. Such transactions have an important function in strengthening the bonds of the family as something with a life beyond that of any individual.

If an older person has assets in terms of a property or money, this too has a function within the family – psychological as well as hard headed. In the past perhaps more than in present-day Britain, older people whose physical strength had waned used their property as a compensatory means of controlling the younger generation, threatening to disinherit those who did not live or marry as the older person desired. These kinds of negotiations undoubtedly still go on, although the laws of the land now limit the absolute freedom of an individual to bequeath away from those who have a claim on the estate and few people depend on land or property as a main source of income. This has not altered the desire of older people to strengthen their family by passing on what they have, however. 'Older home owners are incensed by the thought that they may not be able to hand their hard-won asset to their children because of what they see as the policy requiring them to sell their home to pay for institutional care' (Askham *et al.* 1999). These authors show that the adult children's relationship with their parents' home is not one of clinical separation. They have, in most cases, keys; they come and go; they help with maintenance and 'are seen (by both) as having rights over the use of their parents' home and an expectation of inheriting' (Askham *et al.* 1999).

Whether or not the children expect it or mind about it, however, the important issue to understand is that some parents who are hoping to bequeath will feel diminished when, because of their frailty, they are required to sell their home to pay for care.

A concluding comment on older people's perspectives

Housing in later life can be a source of contentment and satisfaction at a lifetime's achievement. Many people are glad to have a home their families can visit and (if they are owners) that they will be able to leave to their children. Too often, however, these feelings are marred by anxiety about money, about obtaining practical help and about obtaining future services should abilities diminish. Housework, gardening, repairs and decorating are serious major problems. Inability to cope with these tasks may affect the sense of self that is bound up with the home.

Conclusion

This chapter began with the paradox that although housing issues are crucial to thousands of individuals they do not collectively make a great political impact, partly because they are mainly experienced in private. For older people in particular, it is only when their housing concerns reach an interface with a public issue by, for example, causing them to be admitted to hospital, that they become a matter of public concern.

There is a considerable difference in outlook between policy matters and service delivery on the one hand and older people on the other. This divergence is serious. Some differences in perspective are inevitable: national policy makers have to consider the national economic good; local decision makers must weigh up competing priorities; housing managers must work with the resources they have. Accepting these limitations, however, it still seems that the gap between the perspectives of older people themselves about the housing and housing services they need and those who control resources is far too wide, and could be narrowed. One way to achieve this would be to convince the policy makers that taking note of the views of older people would be beneficial to the wider community. Supporting the idea that such rethinking could achieve better value for money is an important theme in the second part of this book.

The size of the challenge should not be underestimated. It strikes at the heart of the idea of 'assessment' for services and at policies focusing resources on 'those in greatest need'. Achieving change would require major shifts in attitude; this is especially hard for those who have been trained to think in these ways and become accustomed to the power such systems give them. There were, however, at the start of the twenty-first century, signs of change.

4

Housing, health and community care

Since the early 1990s, there has been a growing appreciation of the important contribution that housing and housing organizations can make to the meeting of community care objectives (Means 1999) as well as an increased understanding of the impact of housing upon health and well-being (Burridge and Ormandy 1993; Royal Institute of Chartered Surveyors 1997; Harrison and Heywood 2000). This chapter addresses both these issues. It will begin by describing the development of community care and primary care policies and go on to discuss how and why housing is now seen as central to the implementation of these policy agendas. The second half of the chapter looks at the contribution that good quality and appropriate housing can make to the well-being of older people and conversely the deleterious health impact of bad and inappropriate housing.

Community care and older people

Since the Second World War, policies for frail older people have assumed that most older people prefer to stay in their own homes for as long as possible because they believe that is the best way to maintain their independence (Means and Smith 1998a). However, it was not until the early 1970s that this broad view was backed up by a commitment from government to develop a wide range of support services to help frail older people avoid residential care. The main reason for this seems to have been the age-old concern (referred to in Chapter 1) that families would use the existence of such services as an excuse to withdraw from burdensome informal caring roles. The late 1940s and 1950s saw an extensive debate about whether or not the welfare state was encouraging families to abandon their moral responsibilities to the young and the old (Means and Smith 1998b: Ch. 6). Or as Rudd (1988) put it:

The feeling that the state ought to solve every inconvenient domestic situation is merely another factor in producing a snowball expansion on demands in the National Health (and Welfare) Service. Close observation on domestic strains makes one thing very clear. This is that where an old person has a family who have a sound feeling of moral responsibility, serious problems do not arise, however much difficulty may be met.

(Rudd 1988: 348–9)

However, by the 1970s there was a widespread acceptance that domiciliary services were essential for two reasons. They were needed by those who lacked family carers if they were to avoid residential care (Shanas *et al.* 1968) and their availability was much more likely to persuade informal carers to continue to play the pivotal role in supporting elderly relatives than they were to be used as an excuse to withdraw (Moroney 1976). New services began to emerge (for example night sitting services) and older ones (home care, meals on wheels and so on) began to be available on a more extensive basis, although such developments were constrained from the mid-1970s onwards by growing restrictions on public expenditure initially triggered by the oil and sterling crises of the early to mid-1970s (Lowe 1999).

Nevertheless, something close to a consensus emerged about the desirability of staying in your own home compared to any form of institutional care, the pivotal assumption being that institutions such as residential homes and nursing homes lack the capacity to be a home. All three authors of this book have contributed in various ways to the literature on staying put (see for example Oldman 1988; Means 1997a, 1997b; Heywood *et al.* 1999) and its potential positive impact upon independence and well-being. At times, there has perhaps been a tendency within this literature to make sweeping assumptions about the inevitable strengths of staying put and the hopeless disadvantages of all forms of communal living. This issue was a key theme in Chapter 2 and is developed further in Chapter 7.

However, for the purposes of this chapter we need only to note the strength and all persuasive nature of this policy assumption combined with a continuing failure to develop an adequate range of support services in the community which would help to ensure the successful implementation of the policy. Indeed policy weaknesses went deeper than even this for two major reasons. First, the policy emphasis may have been on living at home but community care policy and practice in the 1970s and early 1980s continued to ignore the crucial issue of the house and its neighbourhood and whether this strengthened or undermined the capacity of the older person to stay put irrespective of the level of support available from relatives and the state. Was the house in disrepair? Was it affordable? Did it need adapting as frailty and impairment increased? Was the house in a high crime area? Such questions were nearly always completely ignored by health and welfare professionals working with older people.

Second, changes to benefit regulations in the early 1980s made it easier for low income residents of private and voluntary homes to claim their fees from the social security system. The fact that this subsidy was based on an assessment of financial entitlement only and not on the need for such care encouraged an explosion of homes in the independent sector. Places rose from 46,900 in 1982 to 161,200 in 1991 and expenditure on social security payments for such individuals had reached a massive £1872 million per annum by May 1991 (Means and Smith 1998a: ch. 3). Government policy favoured care in the community – the reality was a massive public subsidy sucking people into residential and nursing home care.

Such a situation could not continue. In December 1986, the then Secretary of State for Social Services asked Sir Roy Griffiths 'to review the way in which public funds are used to support community care policy and to advise me on the options for action that would improve the use of these funds as a contribution to more effective community care' (Griffiths 1988: iii). The resulting Griffiths Report (1988) and the subsequent White Paper on *Caring for People: Community Care in the Next Decade and Beyond* (DoH 1989) were underpinned by three main themes:

- Choice and efficiency needed to be stimulated through a mixed economy approach in which the public, private and voluntary sectors compete to provide services on an equal footing.
- The system of subsidizing independent sector residential and nursing homes through the social security system was wasteful.
- Responsibilities for community care were unclear between health and social services.

The proposed approach (subsequently enabled by the NHS and Community Care Act 1990 and outlined in detailed policy guidance: see DoH 1990) stressed that local authorities rather than health authorities/trusts should have the lead agency role for all the main community care groups including older people. They would be required to produce an annual community care plan in consultation with other key agencies which set out their purchasing intentions and how they were going to maximize the use of the independent sector. At the operational level, the central task was assessment (often called care management) which involved assessing need against eligibility criteria and then pulling together a care package of support from whichever agencies were able to respond to the needs of the client in a flexible, cost-efficient way. Social services authorities were also given the assessment role for those wanting a public subsidy to enter residential or nursing home care as well as the responsibility for then providing that subsidy (a formula was created for transferring the money from the social security budget to individual social services authorities). In this way, the care manager could decide with the client whether their needs were best met through residential care or a care package in their own homes.

This is broadly the community care system which remains in operation at the present time (the impact of primary care changes and debates about pooled budgets between health and social services will be discussed later). This system has been criticized in a number of different ways. The 'new' community care has been seen as hopelessly underfunded and hence denying support for vast numbers of frail elderly people who fail to meet eligibility criteria. Commentators complain that care management has become a form filling, administrative exercise designed to justify the necessary rationing

(Dominelli and Hoogvelt 1996) leading to what some commentators call 'care in chaos' (Hadley and Clough 1996). More recently, Rummery and Glendinning (1999) have pointed out how the new funding system for residential and nursing home care has reduced the rights of people to gain entry to such provision and increased the extent to which they are made to pay for such care, a point broadly supported by the Royal Commission on Long Term Care (Royal Commission 1999). Against this, the Audit Commission (1997) has complained that social services authorities still find it easier to let people drift into residential and nursing home care from hospital rather than provide complex packages of rehabilitation and care at home. Others have complained about the reluctance to explore the scope for preventive services to reduce this drift into hospitals and long-stay provision in the first place (Lewis *et al.* 1999; Phillips *et al.* 1999).

Nevertheless, it can be argued that the existing community care system has helped to provide creative and flexible care packages to at least some frail older people where they are deemed to meet eligibility criteria (Means and Smith 1998a), an outcome which is sometimes referred to as the creation of a Rolls Royce service for the few. There has also been a growing recognition from social services of the central importance of housing and housing organizations to meeting community care objectives, and it is to this subject that we now turn.

Housing and community care

The Griffiths Report (1988) on community care largely ignored housing issues and argued that the responsibilities of housing agencies should be restricted to arranging and sometimes managing the 'bricks and mortar of housing need for community care purposes' (Griffiths 1988: 15). However, the report was widely criticized for its failure to recognize housing and housing policy as one of the foundations of community care (Oldman 1988). The White Paper *Caring for People: Community Care in the Next Decade and Beyond* (DoH 1989) took a much bolder view of the role of housing. 'Suitable good quality housing' was perceived as crucial to care packages and it was argued that 'social services authorities will need to work closely with housing authorities, and other providers of housing of all types in developing plans for a full and flexible range of housing' (DoH 1989: 9). Not only that, but by 1997, central government had provided both detailed strategic (DoH/DoE 1997) and operational guidance (Means *et al.* 1997) on the need for partnerships in community care across housing, health and social services. The centrality of housing was further reinforced by the Royal Commission on Long Term Care with its emphasis that 'the role of housing will be central to the future of long term care' (Royal Commission 1999: 77).

So why did this major change in attitudes come about? Housing organizations had some success in making the point that housing was the essential ingredient of community care. One factor was undoubtedly the impact of the home improvement agency movement ('Care and Repair' and 'Staying Put' projects) in raising the profile of housing issues in later life and their relevance to meeting community care needs. Both the then national co-ordinating agencies (for example Care and Repair England) and a series of individual studies (Harrison and Means 1990; Leather and Mackintosh 1992; Smart and Means 1997) profiled the poor housing of older people and how this might undermine an ability to stay put and, equally, how home adaptation (bathroom alterations, handrails, stair-lifts and so on) could be crucial to enabling someone to remain in their own home.

Second, governments have become very attracted to the potential of sheltered housing, and especially very sheltered housing, as an alternative care environment for frail older people which is alleged to be cheaper than residential care and in which the older person remains a tenant rather than a resident. The perceived potential of these schemes as a cheap and more homely alternative to residential care has been a major factor in the growing influence of housing organizations in community care policy debates. A more detailed discussion of the issues surrounding sheltered housing is presented in Chapter 7.

A third factor behind housing becoming more central to community care, is, therefore, the willingness of housing associations to seek out central government and social services authorities and to argue that they have a crucial role to play in community care on a number of fronts. First, several of them are the managing agents for individual home improvement agencies (HIAs) and they joined the argument that HIAs are so crucial to community care that they required funding from health and social services agencies as well as housing. Anchor Trust, which runs HIAs under the title of Staying Put projects, commissioned a series of studies to back up this claim (Harrison and Means 1990; Smart and Means 1997). Second, housing associations have been at the centre of debates about sheltered housing, both in terms of its capacity to be a home for life (Trotter and Phillips 1997) and in terms of the potential of very sheltered housing schemes to be a direct alternative to residential care. Third, some housing associations have been keen to stress their actual and potential direct provider role in terms of nursing homes, residential homes and domiciliary services (National Federation of Housing Associations (NFHA) 1994). They have been able to present themselves as reliable contributors to the development of a mixed economy of welfare. Finally, housing associations have lobbied central government about the importance of prevention. Until recently, preventive services were seen as unaffordable by central government and individual social services authorities within existing public expenditure limits. As argued earlier in this chapter and in Chapter 3, eligibility criteria were developed to screen out all but those most at risk and most dependent. One consequence of this is that many of the typical tenants of sheltered housing have support needs but not ones which meet the eligibility criteria of the local social services authority, especially given their access to a warden. Housing associations believe that this has unfairly pushed care costs on to them and is short sighted. This is because intervention from social services often comes only after a major life crisis, such as hospital entry, at which point it might be difficult to avoid residential or nursing home entry (Means 1996). With the Joseph Rowntree Foundation, Anchor Trust established a National Preventive Task Group which produces a regular newsletter and has commissioned research (Lewis *et al.* 1999) which defines prevention as having a dual focus:

- services which prevent or delay the need for more costly intensive services
- strategies and approaches which promote the quality of life of older people and their engagement with the community.

The overall prevention message of housing associations to central government has been that a relatively modest investment in prevention services could reduce hospital, nursing home and residential care entry by helping to make ageing in place a reality for most tenants of sheltered housing.

More recently the government's *Supporting People* (DSS 1998b) proposals have helped stress the importance of housing based support services as a credible alternative to more costly community care services. In 2003 a new policy and funding framework will be implemented which will replace the present complex and fragmented system for the funding of housing and support. In so far as the proposals will lead to the expansion of support services, the initiative is to be welcomed but, as Chapter 7 notes, the replacement of the current demand led, entitlement based and mainly social security funded scheme by a cash-limited one administered by local authorities may not in reality lead to the importance of housing support being adequately recognized.

The above analysis of the contribution that housing agencies have made to getting housing on the community care agenda should not be exaggerated. The real push came not from the housing side but from the Department of Health and its various local representatives. It became quickly apparent that the objectives of the new legislation could not be realized without their housing colleagues being 'on side'. The central thrust to the reforms was reducing reliance on costly residential care. Poor and inappropriate housing, it was increasingly seen, was making it harder to keep people at home. As Allen (1997) has so persuasively argued, housing still has a largely technical role to play in community care. Recognizing the importance of housing does not represent, on the part of policy makers, a conversion to genuine principles of independent living which emphasize empowerment and choice. Getting housing on board rather, simply means trying to reduce overall costs by placing more pressures on informal carers. As Chapter 2 has suggested, the focus is on dependency. The corner piece to community care is assessment in which the user is minimally involved and in which housing need is very narrowly defined (Allen *et al.* 1998). Equally the relatively new commitment to a preventive agenda heralded by the Social Services White Paper *Modernising Social Services* (DoH 1998a) is quite silent on the explicit contribution of housing to the agenda. The dialogue between housing organizations and health and social services has focused overly on a new role for sheltered housing and/or the needs of those older people living in the social rented sector. However, the majority live neither in rented housing nor in sheltered housing. Finally, the increasingly strategic approach noticed by Fletcher *et al.* (1999) in their analysis on the emergence of very sheltered housing derives more from a concern with Best Value and achieving better cost effectiveness than a genuine conversion to principles of citizenship and empowerment.

Primary care, the 'new' public health and housing

At first glance, the health policy agenda of the Labour government elected in May 1997 can only help to integrate further the role of housing and housing organizations in community care. The emphasis of this health agenda has been on recognizing the environmental causes of ill health (including housing) and on the need to make health provision driven by primary care with its roots in the community rather than by hospitals. However, there are dangers that this consequent massive organizational change in primary care will disrupt the strong linkages that have begun to develop in most localities between housing and social services.

The Green Paper on *Our Healthier Nation: A Contract for Health* (DoH 1998b) and the subsequent White Paper on *Saving Lives: Our Healthier Nation* (DoH 1999a) both recognized the wide determinants of health and the role that housing can play in it:

> The government recognizes that the social causes of ill health and the equalities which stem from them must be acknowledged and acted on. Connected problems require joined-up solutions. This means tackling inequality which stems from poverty, poor housing, pollution, low educational standards, joblessness and low pay. Tackling inequalities generally is the best means of tackling health inequalities in particular.
>
> (DoH 1998b: 12)

The overall message was the need to tackle the social, economic and environmental factors tending towards poor health but that 'people can make individual decisions about them and their families' health which can make a difference' (DoH 1999: ix). The perceived connections at the individual and macro levels are outlined in Table 4.1 in the next section of the chapter. This new public health agenda was to be driven forward by each health authority producing a published health improvement programme (HIMP) in consultation with social services and other key agencies and backed up by central government setting clear health targets especially in the chosen priority areas of cancer, coronary heart disease and stroke, accidents and mental health.

The government has also been clear that much of this health agenda needed to be delivered through the new primary care arrangements outlined in the earlier White Paper, *The New NHS: Modern and Dependable* (DoH 1997a). This outlined a four stage development of a radical new framework for primary care based upon primary care groups (PCGs) to covering populations of around 100,000. At stage one, the PCG would act as an advisory body to its local health authority which will retain the health care budget. The PCG takes devolved responsibility for budgets in stage two but remains part of the health authority. This changes in stage three when the PCG becomes a primary care trust (PCT) with a budget of at least £60 million and is then a free-standing body accountable to the authority for commissioning care. At stage four, the PCT has added responsibility for providing community services and this is likely to include pooled budgets with social services for much of its community care provision. It is not assumed that all PCGs will get to stage four.

Each PCG has had to establish a board comprised of between four and seven general practitioners (GPs), one of whom is likely to take the chair, one or two community nurses, a local services service representative, a lay member and the appointed chief executive of the PCG. If a PCG becomes a trust, the composition of the board stays the same at stage three but at stage four this changes with a greater emphasis on representation from local nurses and other community and public health professionals.

So why is all of this problematic in terms of enabling the housing dimension of community care to be moved forward? After all, these changes seem to strengthen the hand of housing and housing organizations with its recognition of the deleterious impact of poor housing upon health. The changes also encourage close working between health and social services which must surely be to the advantage of housing. However, the creation of primary care groups and primary care trusts represent a massive programme of organization change (Glendinning and Wilkin 1999) and it is known that this is likely to lead to what policy analysts call 'implementation deficit' (Pressman and Wildavsky 1973). To put it simply, things are likely to get worse before they get better. For example, an enormous amount of energy will need to be invested in board formation and development. It is already known that relationships and linkages are often weak between social services and primary care in general (Hudson 1999) including with regard to older people (O'Hagan 1999). These new changes to structures can only serve to make this even more uncomfortable in the short to medium term even if the long-term agenda is to create structures that better facilitate joint working. For example, in the Avon Health Authority area, six PCGs were originally established but it is now expected that these will need to be reduced to three or possibly only two groups in order to create a viable base for the establishment of primary care trusts. This creates enormous uncertainty for staff. And once trust status has been agreed, these new trusts will need to negotiate with existing NHS trusts about the handover of community health services prior to the completion of stage four. Under these circumstances, it may be difficult for housing to get a look in. However, the most immediate threat to the progress on joint working between housing and care agencies is the fact that housing has not been allowed representation on PCG boards.

Roles and responsibilities have also become muddied. Social services were given the lead agency role in community care but it is far from clear that this will remain the reality after stage four PCT status has been achieved, given the encouragement of government to establish pooled budgets for the commissioning of services across health and social care. Equally, the introduction of health improvement programmes has placed a large question mark over the future of the community care plan which housing organizations are so centrally locked into in most localities. The driving force for community care is shifting to primary care and away from social services, yet housing has much stronger links with the latter (Smart and Means 1997).

All of this means that housing organizations may struggle to keep housing high on the agenda of primary care and public health in the next few years.

However, they have already proved themselves to be effective at the national and local level in raising the profile of housing in community care. These same skills now need to be applied to the health service.

Health and housing

One obvious tactic in attempting to keep housing high profile is to emphasize the strong links between health and housing. These are certainly strong grounds for doing this both in terms of the general population and with regard to older people in particular. However, before this evidence is reviewed it is necessary to offer a short profile of health and ill heath in later life.

A number of authors have criticized the tendency to associate later life with ill health and decline rather than emphasizing the rich possibilities of later years (Wilson 1991; Bytheway 1995). All three authors of this book would support such a position. However, it does still need to be recognized that biological ageing in later life is associated with increased illness, impairment and general frailty, especially once people pass the age of 75. Sidell (1995) reviewed evidence from a range of sources and concluded that the incidence of a limiting long standing illness increases significantly with age as illustrated in Table 4.1. She also indicated that patterns of illness showed some gender differences:

Table 4.1 Percentage of older people reporting long-standing illness

	Women		Men	
	65–74 *n* = 592	75 and over *n* = 344	65–74 *n* = 448	75 and over *n* = 231
Arthritis	17.5	20.0	8.0	7.0
Heart disease	9.5	12.0	12.0	11.0
High blood pressure	8.5	10.5	7.5	7.0
Orthopaedic condition	3.5	4.0	2.5	5.0
Back trouble	4.0	4.0	3.0	1.5
Sight	3.0	4.0	4.0	3.5
Stroke	2.5	3.5	4.0	4.0
Bronchitis	3.0	3.0	5.0	7.0
Diabetes	3.0	2.0	0.5	3.0
Gastric/intestinal	2.0	2.0	2.0	1.0
Depression	2.0	1.5	0.2	–
Thyroid	1.5	1.5	0.2	–
Respiratory disease	1.5	2.0	2.5	3.5
Deafness	1.0	2.5	2.5	3.5
Cancer	1.5	1.5	1.0	1.0
Hernia	1.5	1.5	1.0	2.5
Stomach ulcer	1.5	1.0	2.5	2.0
Anaemia	1.0	1.5	1.5	1.5
Genito-urinal	0.5	2.0	1.0	3.0

Source: Sidell 1995: 44

Many more women than men have arthritis. But also the percentage of women reporting arthritis rises with age whereas for men it decreases. In fact this tendency for women's illnesses to increase with age and for men's to decrease reflects a general trend to all the illnesses. There are some exceptions. For women, diabetes, depression, stomach ulcers, diminish with age. For men, orthopaedic conditions, diabetes, respiratory diseases, deafness, hernias and diseases of the genito-urinary systems increase with age. This indicates that men who survive into old age do not, like the women, tend to accumulate highly symptomatic diseases and conditions.

(Sidell 1995: 45)

Older women over 75, of course, greatly outnumber men of that age; the older population over 75 has widespread chronic health problems, problems likely to be exacerbated by poor and/or inappropriate housing.

However, Sidell (1995) makes the crucial point that it is not the presence or absence of illness *per se* which defines individuals' health and well-being but rather how they cope with these. In general, women cope much better than men with the challenges of ill health. They are better at reconstructing meaning to their life and at drawing upon personal resources, social supports and health care after bereavement or the onset of major illness. It is easy to see how the home, one's housing and the local neighbourhood can all be crucial to the re-establishment of equilibrium after these kinds of eventualities have to be faced in later life.

Three further dimensions of health in later life will now be looked at, namely mental health problems in later life, the health of black and minority elders and the health of homeless people. Numerous studies have shown a high incidence of depression among older people (see Coleman 1994). Although depression is a highly treatable disease, there is evidence that it is often not diagnosed and even when it is, it is often not responded to. One reason for this is believed to be the tendency to equate dementia with mental health problems in old age, with dementia being a progressive illness which shows little if any response to conventional drug treatment.

Dementia is essentially a progressive impairment of cognitive function in a conscious person which is usually untreatable (Wilcock 1990). The term 'dementia' covers a syndrome or collection of symptoms which includes deteriorating memory and reasoning, difficulty with language and recognition, problems carrying out previously familiar tasks and changes in personality. These symptoms can be generated by a range of diseases, the most common of which is Alzheimer's disease. Dementia prevalence does increase with age and approximately 20 per cent of the population over 80 years will have a dementing illness (Jorm and Korten 1988). However, in saying this, it must be stressed that 80 per cent will not.

Until recently, dementia was treated as a medical problem, although one for which there was no cure and little hope. However, there is a growing focus upon the person with dementia and the need to apply a social model of disability which stresses their rights and integrity as humans, and therefore their continued ability to feel and express emotions, and to indicate, where possible, their views about services (Kitwood and Benson 1995; Goldsmith 1996).

Mental health problems can threaten a person's ability to stay in their own home as much as physical health problems. Depression can lead to neglect of the home which may be seen by relatives or social services as a reason to encourage moving to sheltered housing or residential care. Furthermore housing factors can contribute to depression; getting no help with the garden, looking at dirty net curtains all day, living in a dangerous neighbourhood can all add to people's sense of hopelessness. However, as already indicated, depression is treatable and home moving may be entirely the wrong 'solution' for the older person. Even more obviously, dementia threatens the ability of a person to stay in their own home, although the emphasis of the government upon care in the community combined with demographic changes seems to ensure that many more people with dementia will do so in the future. This raises some big issues about the capacity of new technology to help older people live in ordinary housing in safety, although such technologies can also raise issues about whether some forms of surveillance infringe the rights of older people (see also Chapter 6). Research by Kitwood *et al.* (1995) suggests older people with dementia can remain comfortably in sheltered housing under certain conditions. First, the older person must have been in the scheme some time and so be known to the tenants. Second, the warden must be fully supported by their agencies and involved in terms of the delivery of any care package from health and social services. Third, both the warden and the other tenants need clear information about dementia.

There has been much written and discussed about the health of black and minority elderly people and the extent to which their patterns of mortality and morbidity differ from the majority elderly population. Blakemore and Boneham (1994: 93) warn that 'it seems important not to treat older black people as exotic specimens of ageing among whom there are completely distinctive patterns of health and disease'. However, their review of the research evidence does lead them to conclude that 'in terms of common illnesses such as cardio-vascular disease or in terms of "ageing problems" the health of older black people is not as good as might be expected' (Blakemore and Boneham 1994: 99). They stress there is no simple non-controversial explanation for this situation but that poverty, arduous work experiences, poor housing and other environmental/structural factors were likely to have been important, as was the slowness of the health service to respond effectively to the needs of multiracial Britain. What is clear is that the combination of poor housing and poor health can create very stressful situations for many black elders, especially given their concerns about the likelihood of experiencing racism if they move to white-dominated sheltered housing or residential care. More recent work by Blakemore (2000) has shown this is especially likely to be true of the Pakistani and Bangladeshi communities.

Finally we turn to health and older homeless people, which further illustrates the complexity of what causes ill health. Are low-income older people in bad health likely to become homeless? Or does homelessness make people ill? The inevitable answer as confirmed by Crane (1999) is a mixture of the two. For example, in terms of mental health problems:

The associations between mental health, stress and homelessness are intricate. For some older people with histories of mental health problems, their illness was only a background factor and had no obvious influence on their becoming homeless. But for others, it interacted with poor daily living skills and vulnerability to produce various pathways into homelessness.

(Crane 1999: 82)

However, Crane also graphically illustrates how life on the street for older homeless people generates depression and despair as well as exacerbating a wide range of health problems. This is bringing us back to the issue of the impact of housing (and sometimes the lack of it) upon health.

Housing and health in later life

As already indicated it is almost impossible to show a clear causal link between bad housing and ill health largely because of the 'confounding variables' problem; it is almost impossible to separate out housing from such linked factors as poverty and poor diet (Burridge and Ormandy 1993). Marsh *et al.* (2000: 412) have pointed out that 'in addition, the effects of poor housing in health may be indirect or take several years to manifest itself'. In other words, an older person with respiratory problems in good quality sheltered housing may be suffering from their poor housing of the past (or perhaps a complex mixture of poor housing, bad working conditions and heavy smoking). However, it is certainly possible to talk in terms of poor housing and the problems of cold, dampness and condensation as being associated with a wide range of health problems.

A wide range of sources has been drawn upon by a number of summary reports (Royal Institute of Chartered Surveyors 1997; Anchor Trust 1998; Health and Housing 1998) to argue that:

- treating illnesses caused by bad housing may cost the NHS £2.4 billion a year
- the remedying of damp and cold housing could save the NHS £800 million per year
- rough sleepers die at an average age of 42
- cold kills at least 30,000 people in their own home every year.

The importance of bad housing was recognized by the Acheson Report (1998) into health inequalities which made a number of recommendations in this area. These included the need for increased availability of social housing for the less well off and improved insulation and heating systems in new and existing buildings, in order to reduce fuel poverty. It also called for an amendment of housing and licensing conditions, and housing regulations on space and amenity to reduce accidents in the home, and asserted the need for policies which reduce the fear of crime and violence, and create a safe environment for people to live in.

Although there are few studies specifically on the impact of bad housing upon older people, the relevance of the above is all too easy to see. Health authorities and other health care agencies are only just beginning to recognize the importance of tackling this dimension of health need and health inequality. However, there is some evidence that both health and social services are starting to recognize the need to fund housing related projects through joint investment funds. Fletcher *et al.* (1999) looked at fifty joint investment plans and found that fifteen of these had an explicit housing dimension, even though the majority of initiatives related to the development of very sheltered housing as an alternative to residential care. Progress, however, is generally slow and Harrison and Heywood's two-year study on the links between housing and the health of older people makes depressing reading: 'the housing and housing services needs of older people are not being addressed systematically through any of the mainstream planning processes associated with health, housing and community care' (Harrison and Heywood 2000: 35).

Harrison and Heywood argue that the opportunity to utilize the expertise of primary care workers in noticing and acting upon the adverse impact of housing on older people's health is continually being wasted. They call for a new role for directors of public health. The latter should be required to produce annual data and performance sets which illustrate the extent to which local housing conditions are affecting the health of older people. Such a development could be pivotal in ensuring recent health policy reforms in primary care and public health work to the full advantage of other people.

There have been a limited number of innovative schemes. Avon Health Authority, for example, has funded a scheme by Care and Repair Bristol to run a hospital discharge project from a recognition that an ability to return home is often restricted by housing problems. Another collaborative possibility is through the involvement of housing organizations in Health Action Zones which are multi-agency partnerships designed to harness the energy of local communities who are experiencing health inequalities. They are based on the belief that long-term planning and an holistic view of health spanning structural issues and individual health choices represents the best opportunity for overcoming such pockets of health deprivation. As explained in *Saving Lives: Our Healthier Nation* (DoH 1999a: 127), they 'are imaginative new ways of providing services which cross boundaries between organizations'. Eleven such zones were established in April 1998 and a further eleven in April 1999, covering both urban and rural areas. As the then National Federation of Housing Associations (NFHA 1994: 2) has argued, '"independent social landlords" (i.e. housing associations) have expertise in involving local communities in decision making and encourage proper consideration of wider social and environmental factors'.

Conclusion

The overall conclusion of this chapter has to be that some progress has been made in recognizing the housing dimension of community care but very little in responding to the connections between health and housing. The central problem, as other chapters of the book have pointed out, is that housing is narrowly defined. It is seen as largely the technical backdrop to community care. It is housing not home which is the focus. Home is, however, much more than bricks and mortar; it is social relationships, it is space both physical and psychological and it is identity. Home and housing should be at the heart of the new preventive agenda but there is little evidence that they are. Community care itself is underfunded and the preventive agenda insufficiently holistic.

PART II

Reporting empirical studies

5

To move or not to move: housing decisions in later life

In Lillehammer, Norway, there is a folk museum of reconstructed habitations and settlements – spread out over a hillside and allowing the visitor to understand how life was lived in Scandinavia in past centuries. One of the striking characteristics of some farmhouses is the inclusion of an elders' house – a smaller house on the same central plot built for the oldest members of the family to move into when younger members took over the main duties of the farmhouse, and used thereafter according to changing needs. These elders' houses are so charming and beautiful that they invoke in the visitor an immediate desire to move in – and envy at a system so practical, seamless and sensitive. The contrast with the difficulties about moving faced by older people in our modern British society is very striking. Where in twenty-first century Britain are the habitations for older people so tempting that younger people wish they could be the ones moving in? Why has the question of making a move as you get older become a source of anxiety for many? In what ways (if at all) does a move in later life differ from other life-course moves, and how could the process be improved? This chapter seeks to answer these questions: to consider what is different about moving in later life; to look at the push and pull factors causing people to move or stay put, the structural issues behind these factors and the options and support systems available whatever choice they make. It will draw heavily on the findings of an 'Innovation and Good Practice' project called HOOP (description below). Finally, it will describe the HOOP methodology, which has been developed to help older people to make these choices – and which could also be used by planners to identify and provide for housing and housing services that are needed but do not exist.

Housing Options for Older People: (the HOOP project)

Between 1997 and 1999, two projects, funded first by Anchor Housing Trust and then by the Housing Corporation, set out to devise and use a technique that would help older people trying to decide whether or not to move (see Heywood *et al.* 1999 for a full account). The principle was to produce a balanced holistic assessment of an individual's housing situation which would show the good points, the problems and the person's priorities. On the basis of this diagnosis, the options available to the person for improving their situation could be discussed and information about possible moves or help with repairs could be supplied. The methodology was tried out between 1997 and 1999 in a collaboration between the University of Bristol, the University of the West of England and a national charitable organization, the Elderly Accommodation Counsel (EAC). EAC provides information from a national database of residential and sheltered accommodation to people who are considering moving into such accommodation or, quite often, to their relatives. All the researchers shared a concern that moves late in life should be well considered, and that information given should be based on a full understanding of the enquirer's circumstances, concerns and priorities.

There is a rich literature on the subject of older people moving (or not moving) home. It includes considerations of statistics, motivation, opportunities, constraints and outcomes, always with a view to ways in which the moves made in later life relate to the life course and are therefore different from those made at other stages. Much of the literature lies within the disciplines of social gerontology and social policy and therefore focuses more on the pathology of later life than on the fine detail of the housing issues. It is the purpose of this chapter to build on the work that has gone before but to pay particular attention to work which emphasizes the housing aspects.

Proportions of people moving

As people get older in Britain, they are less likely to move home. A survey in 1989 found that 70 per cent of people aged 55–64 and 73 per cent of those aged 65 or more had not moved for ten or more years, compared with 45per cent of those aged 35–54 (Coles 1989: 15). Statistical information for the Office for National Statistics adds to this information. In their survey of 1995–6 (ONS 1997: table 1.15) it is shown how the likelihood of moving goes down steadily with age. In all, only 8 per cent of over-60s who were heads of household had moved in a three year time span compared with 32 per cent of those under 60 (Leather 1999: 32–7).

The largest number of moves by older people in 1991–4 were made by owner-occupiers moving into alternative owner-occupied properties. However, 37,000 older owners in this period (16 per cent of all those who moved) had moved into council or housing association rented property; a further 10,000 had moved into private renting. Those older people who had moved *out of* private rented accommodation (68,000 in the three years to 1994) had moved primarily into social rented housing. The number of older renters who moved into owner occupation was minimal, though the statistics do not include those who changed tenure without moving by exercising their right to buy. What they do show is the importance of a social rented sector as an option for older people as it was the only sector where there was a net gain in numbers.

To complement the information on changes between tenure, Leather draws on the 1991 census to show the geographical patterns of older people's house moves. It will not surprise many readers to learn that the areas into which older people were least likely to have moved were large urban areas. Nineteen out of the twenty authorities with the lowest numbers of older in-migrants were London boroughs. Authorities with the highest proportion of in-migration of pensioner households included Milton Keynes and Winchester, besides the more predictable areas of the West Country, Gloucestershire and rural and seaside areas in the north, east and south (Leather 1999: 36).

This statistical information is a useful starting point, though more detail would be needed to understand its significance. The moves into private renting, for example, will have included people moving into up-market flats or sheltered housing as well as those studied by Hawes (1997) who lost their homes through repossession, divorce or family conflict in old age and were forced into poor quality private renting. Similarly, low migration into London boroughs may indicate that older people do not want to move into London, or it may indicate that there are no properties into which they could move, because of high house prices and shortage of housing to rent. It is not possible to understand the moving patterns without knowing a lot more about the housing situation as well as about the preferences of those who moved or chose not to move. These particular statistics do not include information about older people who moved in with family, or into residential accommodation. They also cannot tell us the reasons behind the moves that were made; how many other people would have moved if suitable options had been available or how many of those who did move felt under pressure to do so or were unhappy with the outcome.

Understanding moves

Social gerontologists have long been interested in moves to residential care. Some have continued the tradition of Booth and Townsend in seeking the experiences of those who have moved into residential accommodation, asking how and why they came to move. What is relevant to this chapter from this school of research is all it has to say about the process of moving and the decision making that precedes it. The focus is primarily on increasing dependency, inability to manage at home and risk of accident. Allen *et al.* (1992: 157–96) present the voices of all the players in such moves including GPs, family members, hospital staff, social workers and the people themselves. The detailed case studies include several sharp reminders that the independence of some people in their eighties and nineties is bought at a very high price to relatives in their sixties and seventies, who give up all their own independence in order to care for the older person.

One factor that is important to the methodology discussed in the later part of this chapter is that Allen *et al.* (1992) found that 77 per cent of the older people interviewed who had moved into residential care had had the idea of moving suggested to them by someone else. 'I fell twice more and the GP said I couldn't stay there if I fell so often. He said the Medical Association didn't allow it' (Allen *et al.* 1992: 159). Some said they had not discussed the move and had not wanted to, but 30 per cent felt that they had not talked the move through with anyone sufficiently before they made it (Allen *et al.* 1992: 169–71). The research also showed that the people concerned had generally had neither many options nor much opportunity to exercise any choice. It was, indeed, in response to this common dilemma for both older people and their relatives that the national charity the Elderly Accommodation Counsel was set up, as a means of supplying information and increasing the possibility of choice.

In the broader sphere of older people moving home there is another body of work which has studied patterns and typologies of move. Bond *et al.* (1993) have considered the patterns of migration in later life as part of a general trend in Europe. Their typology is that people must have both the resources and the desire to move and that the deciding factor will be whether social networks encourage or discourage a move (Bond *et al.* 1993: 207–8). Bond and the other authorities he cites observe that older people's migration is something that happens principally at the time of retirement (see also Karn 1977). They suggest that it is chiefly the prerogative of people from middle or upper income groups. Even the growing trend of migration of older people from northern European countries to the poorer countries of the Mediterranean (Warnes 1991) consists mainly of such income groups.

Bond does not show much awareness of housing factors in this typology but the same is not true of Burholt, another social gerontologist. Burholt's (1997) own work focused on a longitudinal study of moves by older people into rural North Wales. In this study, typologies of moving developed by Litwak and Longino (1987) and Wiseman (1980) were tested and the Wiseman model adapted to produce a typology that had fewer categories but accurately captured the variety of motives affecting relocation or non-relocation given by people in the case study. Litwak and Longino (1987) had classified motives for moving in later life as 'retirement', 'moderate disability' and 'major chronic disability'. Burholt (1997) found these categories inadequate to fit the data. She found a much better fit with her adaptation of Wiseman's original eight categories to five:

- long-distance amenity
- wide choice local amenity
- narrow choice local amenity
- low levels of assistance
- high levels of assistance.

Burholt points out that the evidence from the people interviewed showed a richer and more varied number of reasons for moving than the classifications by themselves could ever capture and stressed the need for qualitative data to enhance understanding. Factors affecting the decision to move or not to move were:

- the reticence or inability to expend the physical and mental energy required to undertake a move
- community ties and social networks
- material culture and attachment to home
- enforced decision making in a confining relationship
- lack of available alternative housing
- perceived suitability of alternative housing.

These are useful categories in thinking about moves in later life, very similar to those within the methodology given below.

In allied but different disciplines, the debate about older people moving home has centred around three related issues: housing satisfaction, the role of sheltered housing, and the community care debate, with its emphasis on maintaining people in their own homes.

Housing satisfaction

In their work entitled *Factors Influencing Housing Satisfaction among Older People*, Wilson *et al.* (1995) present a summary of the approaches to this subject that have been influential in planning housing for older people. Disengagement theory, for example, has been used to explain older people's perceived indifference to their housing conditions. It supposedly shows why high satisfaction scores are given for objectively poor housing. We would argue, however, that these findings probably say more about the poor quality of housing satisfaction surveys than they do about older people's views (Heywood 1997). Wilson *et al.*'s (1995) reanalysis of a survey of 1557 older people in a range of housing in Scotland has been valuable in dispelling some of the myths that long surrounded the issue of housing satisfaction and older people. They found no clear relationship linking levels of satisfaction with increasing age. They found that damp was easily the best predictor of housing dissatisfaction and that people who had moved within the previous five years were more likely to be satisfied or very satisfied than those who had been in their homes ten years or more. Some caution is needed here, as people who move late in life and are unhappy may die, and therefore not be available to give their views, but the evidence certainly shows that there are old people who are not happy with their homes and might like to move.

Oldman (2000a) has also challenged received wisdom about older people's satisfaction with their housing. Qualitative interviews in Middlesbrough with a random and varied sample showed the disabling effect of much of the housing occupied, and that a significant number of owner-occupiers wanted to leave the tenure. Oldman's (1991b) work on the financial effects of moving in old age has shown, however, the constraints that may prevent people moving. These barriers include not only the costs of moving but also the disincentives of the benefits system that mean owners in receipt of income support who sell their home and move into rented property stand to erode their capital, as they will cease to receive benefit until their capital has been reduced to the limit allowed by government (£16,000 at the time of writing). Most significantly of all, Oldman found that, where there were service charges as well as rent, many of those who had moved were paying out considerably more in housing costs than they had previously paid. Some of those interviewed felt that the benefits of being in safe secure housing, free of worries, outweighed the increased costs but it is important to note that moving may or may not result in lower housing costs. What is even more important is the study's finding that 'the main reason for not moving was the perception that they could not afford to do so' (Oldman 1991b: 261).

The question of sheltered housing

Much of the debate about moves in later life has centred round the issue of whether or not 'sheltered' housing is a desirable form of provision. Caution and a sense of proportion are necessary here because such a small percentage of older people live in sheltered housing, but it is obviously important to know whether more such provision is required and whether its absence is preventing people from moving. Chapter 7 shows that the growth of sheltered housing stalled in the 1980s in a political climate of 'targeting' resources, and following research (Butler *et al.* 1983; Clapham and Munro 1988) that questioned whether those moving in really needed the level of support offered. Critics also suggest that sheltered housing does not fit well with a social model of ageing and creates ghettos of older people isolated from the rest of the community. What has emerged in subsequent research is the understanding that people who move to sheltered housing are more interested in its housing characteristics (secure, accessible, no responsibilities for maintenance or gardening) and the perceived social aspects, than they are in the 'support' services, except for an alarm system for emergencies. It may also be worth suggesting that older people's wishes should carry considerable weight in this debate.

Moving in old age and the great community care debate

The community care policies introduced through the NHS and Community Care Act 1990 were like a building constructed without foundations. Everything about the new approach rested on the notion of older people living in their own housing rather than in institutions. The backlash by policy makers against sheltered housing in the 1980s was part of the whole finance-driven community care debate that culminated in the new Act. Although sheltered housing is not residential care, it was caught up in the same web when the emphasis, in rhetoric at least, was on policies of Staying Put. Obviously, if there was an assumption that older people wanted to stay in their own homes, there was no need to plan provisions to enable them to move, which is why the community care debate is so fundamental to the topic of this chapter. Figures given at the end of this chapter for the drop in new housing provision show how seriously this debate has affected housing options for older people. Failure to provide for the housing aspects of community care has created problems for older people. Harrison and Heywood (2000) conclude that this policy vacuum has been possible politically because the problems are invisible, concealed in the privacy of many individuals' homes.

Oldman probably sums up the moving/not moving debate as it stands at the time of writing when she says, simply, 'It cannot be always assumed that older people do not want to move' (Oldman 2000a: 18). Here in this book we are no longer assuming that older people are indifferent to cold, damp, unadapted housing; instead we are recognizing that people move or stay put chiefly for housing reasons, which need to be better understood. The next section, which presents Heywood and authors' of this chapter's analysis of the issues of moving in later life, is based in an ethnographic approach, using both the work done by others in listening to the views of older people and incorporating material coming out of the HOOP project.

Moving in later life: some characteristics

The retirement dream move

Many people, while they are at work, long for the day when they are no longer tied (to their children's schools or their job in the town) and can move at last to somewhere more peaceful and pleasant in the country or by the sea – where land and housing are cheaper, the air is cleaner and the scenery more pleasant. Many people achieve such a move in their late fifties or early sixties and are happy to have done so. Nor is this a trend confined to the affluent middle classes. One route is the purchase or rental of a mobile home, and many older people choose to house themselves in this way. The Greater London Council, before its abolition, set up a 'bungalows by the sea' scheme: building or buying properties in seaside resorts so that tenants over 60 could move out of London boroughs. The scheme still exists in the year 2000. Its 3000 properties have been transferred to housing associations but their allocation is managed for all the London boroughs by the Seaside and Country Homes Agency, which is answerable to the DETR. Large housing associations may also offer their city tenants a move from, for example, Leeds to Bridlington or Scarborough. The large proportion of residents of pension-able age in seaside areas (Christchurch 34.6, East Devon 31.5, Colwyn 27.9 per cent) compared with the national average of 18.7 per cent (Office of Population Census and Surveys (OPCS) 1994) testified to this trend. (For the statistics given for the 1991 census, 'pensionable age' meant women of 60+, men of 65+.)

It is a subject that was studied in depth in the 1970s by Valerie Karn (1977) in her work *Retiring to the Seaside*. She showed that retirement communities (not necessarily by the sea) have existed since Roman times, and that, in the twentieth century, the high percentage of retired residents in British seaside towns was replicated all along the coastlines of France, Spain and Portugal. Her detailed study of people who had retired to Bexhill or Clacton concluded that such moves were generally very successful. Those who moved before or just after retirement settled more happily than those who moved later, and people who had always been single fared better than those who became widowed after the move. In general however, people were well pleased with their moves and rarely expressed regret. The people in the study felt that they benefited from being in a town which was well geared to the needs of their age group, rather than also-rans in a commuter suburb. The major problem noted was the failure of health and social services to provide services in proportion to need. Karn's study also supports the generalized finding that part of what is hard about moving is the change of status from 'resident' to 'newcomer', but that this is more tolerable in situations where many others are also newcomers (Steinfeld 1981: 206).

Immigrants who have spent their working lives in Britain also often dream of retiring home – to the West Indies or Ireland or India. Every year some do so, and again, for some it works and for others not. People may find that the country to which they return is not the one they left: the very money they and others have sent back may have caused serious changes in the social structure – and once more the ability to adapt may be the key to a chance of happiness.

There are disadvantages to retiring to a rural or seaside area in Britain, too. If one partner dies soon after such a move, the other (especially if their partner drove and they do not) may find themselves isolated. The winters may be oppressive, as can be the absence of younger people. But there are also many advantages, and how 'the dream' works out may depend largely on individuals' disposition and expectations. These moves made at or around the point of retirement are important but are not the main focus of this chapter.

How does moving house in old age differ from moving at other stages in the life course?

The explanations about why a move in later life may be different are rooted in theories about the meaning of home. Gurney's hierarchy for the meanings that are attached to someone's home was presented in Chapter 2 (Gurney and Means 1993: 126). Some meanings are culturally determined (Knightsbridge seen as more desirable than Peckham). Some are entirely personal (this is the tree that I planted; the place where I composed my masterpiece). In between will be a range of factors affecting meaning which are neither cultural nor personal (for example, noise from a newly built motorway, access to transport and shops) which Gurney calls 'intermediate'. This hierarchy of meanings serves to remind us how complex the issue is and how an individual will not have control over the cultural or intermediate factors. Someone who moved into a sought-after council home forty years ago, for example, and who has maintained it in pristine condition ever since, may find the meaning or value they used to attach to their housing under assault from the culture of owner-occupation, from the sudden collapse of employment in the area or from deteriorating standards on their estate. At all three levels – personal, intermediate and cultural – a person is liable to identify themselves with their home and make a judgement about both together. This is more likely when someone has lived in one place a reasonable length of time and more likely when a great deal of work has gone into the making of a home, but it is not a product of old age as such. In our view, the meaning of home is not qualitatively different in later life. What is difficult about so many moves in old age is that there is a danger they will be seen by others as signifying a loss of status and independence.

At the cultural level, for example, in a society which equates 'bigger' with 'better' and owning as somehow superior to renting, the moves many older people make (larger to smaller; owning to renting) are likely to be seen as a 'downward step' when all previous moves have been 'upward'. It often signifies what both older people and others see as a negative status passage in the life cycle, for example, loss of income, loss of a partner, loss of health (Gurney and Means 1993: 123). Younger people who have to move to lower status homes because of repossession or compulsory purchase experience the same kind of distress. 'We call this loss of home, loss of job, our big tragedy' (Heywood and Naz 1990: 159). Steinfeld (1981) concludes that if existing housing symbolizes a valued identity, people will probably choose not to move, but they will if the housing no longer supports the maintenance of that identity. Importantly, he points out that in the case of disadvantaged older people, society may make the decision. The age-segregated provision they are then offered may restrict their chances to participate in majority culture and so contribute to a devalued image of older people (Steinfeld 1981: 242).

At the personal level, a move in later life may signify a role reversal with adult children, the children taking on the 'parent' role as the older people move to be near them or move at their suggestion. Finally, a move in old age may be forced when all other moves have been voluntary. In short, moving in later life may threaten a person's status in society, their position in the family and their autonomy. Such major challenges may help to explain why many older people decide not to move. This is not to deny, of course, that some moves may be extremely positive and improve status and confidence, especially if something dramatic like a move to Portugal or the West Indies is involved.

The anticipatory move and the forced move

Ambitions and dreams apart, there are two kinds of moves which people make specifically because of the changing circumstances that are caused by increasing age, and these moves are the core subject of this chapter. Oldman (1990: 52) summed up the key points and work on the HOOP project reinforced her findings. In the one instance, people plan a move in advance to somewhere more manageable, accessible, cheaper or safer so that whatever happens, they will be well prepared; and, in the other, a sudden and traumatic life event forces a move upon them. Discussion with older people shows that the first of these processes is something people may consider over a very long period – perhaps 20–30 years – before they act. One woman interviewed for the HOOP project said she had decided in her early eighties that she would move nearer to her daughter when she was 90 (which, subsequently, she did).

Whether someone has been a single parent in a two-bedroomed flat or a couple in a three- or four-bedroomed house, why should they feel a need to move when their children leave home and they gain an extra room?

Very few people think they have too much space (see Heywood 1993: 21) and most like to have a room for visitors, even if visitors are infrequent. Wilson *et al.*'s study of factors influencing housing satisfaction among older people also found that few people in the sample felt they were living in a house that was too large for their needs (Wilson *et al.* 1995: 11). But there comes a time when other factors begin to weigh.

Push factors: driving people out

Table 5.1 lists some of the negative factors about their housing (landlord pressure apart) which may cause older people to want to move out. The text that follows discusses some of the points in more detail.

Lower income, higher costs

For most people, retirement brings a reduction in income, which will go on reducing steadily the older they become. In 1998, when the average disposable weekly household income in the UK was £371, it was £249 for those aged 65–74 and £182 for the over 75s. Single pensioners mainly dependent on the state pension had an average disposable income of £97 (ONS 1999a: 8.1, 8.2). For those over 80 most of whom are women the situation was worse still. About 25 per cent lived on £80 per week or less (Milne 1999). At the same time, if people are at home most of the day, their heating costs will inevitably rise, all the more so as they become less mobile and need a higher ambient temperature in the house in order to keep warm. Other costs will rise too. If you can no longer safely do your own decorating, gardening, housework or maintenance jobs, you will either have to wait for relatives to help or pay for what you would once have done yourself.

Financial effects of bereavement

These problems of reducing income and rising costs are hard enough for a couple, but the final blow may come when one person in a shared household dies. Overheads for a single person may be almost as high as they are for a

Table 5.1 Factors pushing older people to move

• Housework problematic	• Garden problematic
• Maintenance problems	• Disrepair
• Cold and damp	• High costs
• Too far from family	• Inaccessible baths
• Problems with stairs	• Crime or fear of crime
• Loneliness, after bereavement	• Anxiety about ability to cope in case
• No longer being able to drive	of accident or illness
• Neighbour nuisance	• Not wishing to become burden on
	friends or relatives

Source: Heywood *et al.* 1999, reproduced by kind permission of the publishers

couple. Council tax is lower, but standing charges for water, telephone, gas and electricity will be the same and needs for heating may actually increase. The costs of maintaining the house itself will not reduce, either, but will have to be paid for from, often, very much reduced income. These financial issues alone put great pressure on widowed older people to move and many anticipate such problems of bereavement by moving before it happens.

Crime and fear of likely crime

Another key issue is crime. Studies of moves into sheltered housing have found that they quite commonly follow a burglary, or that fear of crime is given as a strong reason for the move (Toffaleti 1997: 13).

Fear of falling

People, especially those who live alone, are also afraid of accidents – of lying on the floor and not being found. Personal alarms have done a lot to allay such fears, but this kind of vulnerability remains a 'push' factor. Steinfeld, quoting a study by Jacobs (1978), concluded that a major motivating factor causing older people to move is the desire for 'security' in the broadest sense of the word (Steinfeld 1981: 206).

Unsuitable design

As people develop the common mobility impairing ailments of old age – rheumatism, arthritis, heart disease – they may find a home with a steep entrance or stairs or steps inside increasingly problematic – especially if the only toilet is up a flight of stairs, or they live in an upper-storey flat with no lift. Less obvious but more serious impediments may be heart disease, or breathlessness, caused by asthma or bronchitis. The stairs and the bath become major design problems for old people, as the plethora of advertisements in over-fifties magazines for stair-lifts and easy-access baths bear witness.

It is common to hear older people worry or plan for what they will do 'when they can no longer manage the stairs'. Some get a new lease of life with the fitting of a second handrail (see Chapter 6). Some plan ahead by fitting a downstairs shower and toilet. Some install a stair-lift, or ask to be assessed for one. But the desire for a home without stairs – a bungalow or a ground floor flat – is another strong incentive to many older people to move. It is not the only design issue – people talk of their homes as inconvenient, hard to clean and decorate, or dark, or chilly – but it is probably the most common.

Other practical issues

The inability to manage housework and gardening, and not wishing to become a burden on relatives, may also be strong incentives to move; research has shown gardening to be perhaps the major issue. The decision to 'give up the car', because of the cost or failing eyesight, may also make a once-loved location very impractical.

Changing neighbourhoods

Noisy or inconsiderate neighbours can drive people of all ages out of their homes, but for housebound older people, or those who sleep badly (as is common in old age), bad neighbours (or even ordinary neighbours, if there are boisterous children, dogs, cats and alarms) can make life a complete misery. Litter and rubbish dropped in common areas, drug dealers and neglect of an environment that was once kept attractive can all be oppressive, as well as noise, to the extent that people feel they must flee.

Loneliness

There is also the overwhelming issue of loneliness, especially after bereavement or when friends die or move away. Crane (1999) reports that some of the homeless older people she interviewed said that the loneliness they experienced after being rehoused was so bad it led them to resume a homeless lifestyle, or start drinking where they had not before. This is extreme, but illustrates what a powerful 'push' factor loneliness may be.

Positive factors: attracting people to move

Some of the positive aspects of a planned move in old age have been discussed above. These and others are listed in Table 5.2. Some of these attractions may be more apparent than real. Loneliness is not necessarily solved by a move to sheltered housing; warden services do not provide the level of support that prospective tenants often expect; and neighbours with poor hearing and loud televisions may drive others in specialized housing to distraction. In one study it was found that whereas only 1 per cent of those waiting for sheltered housing said they would rather have help to stay in their own home, 18 per cent of people already in such housing said they would prefer their own home (Age Concern Scotland *et al.* 1997: 12). Also, the guarantee of care, whatever befalls, is at present confined to a small number of people in experimental retirement villages such as that set up by the Joseph Rowntree Foundation at Hartrigg Oaks near York. Nevertheless it is useful to remember the positive benefits that may come from a move, as so much emphasis is normally placed on staying put.

Table 5.2   Some attractions of moving to alternative accommodation

• No garden (or garden maintained by someone else)	• Care guaranteed, so no further move ever necessary
• More company	• Good access to shops, doctor and so on
• Nearer to relatives	• No stairs
• Less risk from crime	• Lower running costs
• Smaller and more manageable	• Equity release from sale of larger home
• Pleasant views and surroundings	• Support available in case of emergency
• Designed for comfort (heating, bathroom, power sockets, windows)	• Clean and peaceful

Table 5.3 Some factors pulling people to stay in their current homes

• Desire to retain independence	• Retaining status
• Deep attachment to home or garden	• Sense of security within familiar home
• Sense of achievement within home	• Comfort in a place tailored to suit
• Memories associated with home	• Home owned outright
• Fear or dislike of change or the unknown	• Attachment to furniture
• Liking more space than other people consider 'necessary'	• Desire to keep the possibility of family visits
• Cost of moving	• Lack of energy to move

Pull factors: reasons for not wanting to move

Some of the deep-seated reasons why people may want to stay put in their existing homes were described in Chapter 3. Table 5.3 lists common factors, which again are a mixture of practical, financial, personal and emotional issues.

Practical issues

For some people, the very thought of the process of moving – regardless of the desirability of a prospective new home is just too daunting. They feel too old and weary and set in their ways to want to be bothered. Others are attached to their furniture and other possessions and know they would not fit into a smaller dwelling. Others like the size and space they have and do not want to lose it.

Financial issues

If a home is owned outright, or someone is a secure tenant, they will feel that any move may increase their outgoings and/or reduce their security of tenure, apart from the actual cost of moving.

Personal and emotional issues

These are much harder for older people to articulate and may make them seem unreasonable to younger people who want them to move. On the issue of poor house condition for example: 'I know it's old, it's damp and my roof wants doing – it leaks. It is in a mess. I can't afford to pay for it, but I'm not going to leave it . . . I've always lived in it' (Mrs P, aged 85, quoted in Gurney and Means 1993: 125).

People come to identify with their homes – and to see them as symbolizing achievement and family history. They see the risk that a move from a large owned house to a small rented flat may diminish them in the eyes of society, or may suggest they are choosing to withdraw. An American study showed how those moving into apartments in a block designated for older people asserted themselves by positioning their best furniture and possessions in the most public place – the lobby or the first room to which strangers might have access, even when this resulted in cramped conditions (Steinfeld 1981: 207). This is a manifestation of the instinct that is in us all, as we put up photographs in the office or otherwise set out to maintain our control over any small piece of territory where we are temporarily abiding.

Independence

Finally, we return to the issue of independence (already covered at some length in Chapter 3). To retain a home of your own is to retain your independence. In that place, you decide on the wallpaper, the temperature, the times of meals and what to watch on the television. If you want to eat Mars bars for breakfast and live on brown ale the rest of the time, let your dog sleep in your bed or cultivate a garden to attract butterflies, you may do so. If you want to endure cold and hunger in order to have more to give your children or grandchildren, that is your choice. However, a move in later life may enhance independence rather than reduce it: Oldman and Quilgars (1999: 376–7) give examples of people who felt they had been growing too dependent on their children, and had restored the balance by moving into housing and care provision.

In Chapter 3 the issue of the changing relationships with children was considered. The role of children in persuading their parents to move is known to be significant (Allen *et al.* 1992: 169) and the corollary of this is the independence some older people assert by deciding not to move, despite the views of their relatives. It is a very hard decision to make, and hard for all parties to be honest about their motives. (Do the children just want peace of mind? Are the parents being selfish?) It is for this reason – because the decision of whether to move house or not in later life is so important yet so difficult – that a methodology which will be described in the remainder of this chapter has been evolved to help the process.

The HOOP approach

The starting point of the HOOP approach was in fact an earlier research project which was not focused on life-course related moves but on 'slum' clearance. If houses are being cleared because they have been judged to be 'unfit for human occupation' as statutorily defined, the occupants will be offered compensation and offers of rehousing. In a study carried out in Birmingham in 1988–9, Heywood and Naz (1990) found that while some of those who experienced this process thought that the move from cold, damp housing had saved their lives, others felt that the change was detrimental overall.

The HOOP methodology was devised because the researchers believed that help was needed to improve the system whereby older people made housing decisions. They knew that some decisions were made at times of crisis and others on the basis of poor information, or under pressure from relatives, landlords or hospitals. They knew that such decisions (especially, but not only, decisions to move) were very difficult to reverse once made, but could be disastrous for the individuals concerned. They believed that sometimes the older person themselves acted without sufficient thought or knowledge and sometimes agencies made assumptions and gave advice in response to a presenting problem, without always checking the whole picture. For example, if the first thing mentioned is disrepair, an enquirer may find themselves swept along the path of renovation, when really they want to move. Or if they begin by saying they think they need a ground floor flat, a landlord (eager for them to vacate a family property) may arrange the move without ever mentioning adaptations as an alternative possibility – and the move may leave the person much worse housed overall. (It may, of course, be very beneficial, but the question needs to be considered.)

The HOOP questionnaire

This is a self-assessment questionnaire, to be filled in at leisure in advance of a discussion with a housing adviser. In the trials it was found that an interviewer was not normally necessary for the completion of the form.

The questions fall into nine categories, reflecting the different aspects of a home which research has shown to be important to older people, and listed in Box 5.1. Within each of these nine categories, respondents first answer some detailed questions and then give a score out of 10 for the category as a whole. This gives an opportunity to air and discuss problems, but also to put them in proportion. For example, in the category 'location', questions include

- Is your home convenient for shops, transport etc.?
- Do you feel safe in the street?
- Is your home a suitable distance from family or friend(s) (however near or far you want to be)?
- Is it as quiet and stress free as you want?

Box 5.1   The Hoop questionnaire

	Score out of 10?	Especially important?
Size and space		
Independence		
Cost (affordability)		
Condition of property		
Comfort and design		
Security		
Location		
Managing		
Quality of life		

One respondent said 'no' to the question about the location being quiet and stress free and discussed neighbour problems at length – but then surprised the interviewer by giving a score of 9 out of 10 for location, indicating that the neighbour problem was in fact largely outweighed by the positive aspects of the location.

The system for scoring out of 10 has a second purpose in the methodology. It is explained to respondents that in choosing a score, they are making a judgement about whether their home is acceptable to them in that category or not. There is a dividing line between '5' and '6' – with '6' being 'Just OK' (that is meeting the person's minimum standard of acceptability) and '5', Just not OK'.

10	9	8	7	6	5	4	3	2	1	0
Perfect				Just OK	Just not OK				Terrible	

When all the categories have been completed and the scores for each are entered on a single chart, there is an at-a-glance representation of what the person likes and dislikes about their home and about where things are so bad that action is needed. A housing adviser who has never met the older person, but who can look at the chart and glance quickly at the nine sections, will begin the interview with a very good holistic view of the person's situation. Besides seeking scores in the nine categories, the HOOP methodology invites respondents to consider their priorities, to look to the future if they wish and to decide whether there is information they need.

The idea of this systematic approach to making housing choices came from researchers, not older people, and the idea is therefore one that has to be 'sold' rather than something which will be seized upon as meeting a strongly felt need. Many older people feel perfectly clear about what they want without filling in a questionnaire and say that they need information about where to find what they want, and practical help with moving, rather than advice about the decision. It was also found to be crucial that the approach was used at the right time – when a person was still wondering what to do not when they had already gone through a long painful decision-making process of their own and had finally made up their mind.

Advantages of HOOP

Many of those interviewed during the project said that what they valued was a chance to talk their situation through with someone and receive, as Harding (1997) recommends in her report for Help the Aged, not just information but advice.

Clarifying thought

Although only a minority of participants said the methodology had helped them to clarify their thoughts, for these few it was valuable. In particular, it helped one woman facing eviction who said the structured format helped her to more reasoned thought where beforehand she had been in a state of panic. Another couple, who had been considering a move into sheltered housing, said that the format had made them realize that they already had as much support as sheltered housing would offer and there was no need to move.

Communicating views to family and professionals

This is perhaps HOOP's greatest strength. Several participants said that completing the form would enable them to explain to a son or daughter why they did not want to move at that time. For advice workers and housing professionals, too, the form can explain a lot quickly, and is helpful to those professionals who are not already experienced and skilled workers. The form empowers older people to stand up to pressure.

Challenging assumptions

Answers given by individuals may constantly surprise. Someone seen by others as a brave and capable manager may use the form to show that she is not managing and that she fears for the future and wants to move. People on a third floor may decide they want to stay there, despite the difficulties. Workers at one day centre for Asian Elders felt that the questions might be culturally inappropriate, and that their old people would not have high expectations about space, privacy or comfort but the interviews given certainly challenged these assumptions.

Room for emotional factors: without intrusion

The HOOP questionnaire allows for recognition of emotional issues in housing decisions, more than an ordinary housing needs assessment form can, but does not intrude or force people to say more than they wish.

Neutrality

The approach is neutral as to staying put or moving. It is designed to encourage in every way possible the person using it to express their own views. This is important because, with the best will in the world, housing agencies where people seek advice may have a stronger interest in some solutions than others.

Detailed diagnosis

Housing providers who are having difficulties in understanding tenant dissatisfaction may use HOOP as a diagnostic tool. One provider, after moving the same tenant several times at his request, discovered through HOOP that the tenant wanted larger rooms than they had in any of their properties. The association then helped him to find a private landlord who could meet his need.

Holistic approach

Above all, this approach is based in a whole view of a person's housing situation, with detailed issues put into a broader context where the bricks and mortar, garden, location, transport and systems of support are all taken into account.

Disadvantages of HOOP

Timing is important if HOOP is to be useful, and for those who reach the point of approaching a housing agency it may be too late. The style of it is not for everyone either, and there is a general tendency for it to be more useful in informing advice givers than it is directly to older people themselves.

The lengthy-looking questionnaire may be off-putting to some people, though in practice it was found to be user-friendly by a wide range of people. There is now a short (one side of A4) version for use in some circumstances.

More problematic than the length to advice givers is the amount of detailed information on need elicited which cannot at present be responded to. People may therefore fear that it will raise expectations which cannot be met. Similarly, the HOOP format may lead people to ask for wide-ranging information, and for advice and support to a high standard. Again expectations will be raised

The future use of HOOP

In the future, it is envisaged that the computerized version of HOOP (already available) could be linked to databases of information (EAC's National Database of Housing for Older People is also already available) to allow people to use the system and discover options in an interactive way from their home, public library or internet café. This approach will not be for all, and should never be considered as an alternative to direct human contact, but could be a supplement. The website, on which all the forms are to be found, is http://www.housingcare.org

It is also felt that the short version could be used in assessing the housing needs of particular populations, or as an adjunct to community care assessment. Both formats contain questions which ask whether any of the different aspects of housing are causing stress or affecting health. There might therefore be a use in conjunction with health planning, including in Health Improvement Areas.

Conclusion

One of the difficulties of using the HOOP methodology described above is that it tends to discover needs which cannot be met. This is but a symptom of the wider issue in our society, which is that in many cases the options that would meet older people's needs do not exist, and the decisions are therefore much harder than they should be. Between 1981 and 1997 the number of new specialized dwellings built per year in England and Wales for older or disabled people went down from 17,000 to 1100 (figures to nearest 100). These figures include all tenures and are for sheltered housing and other housing designated for these groups. It is not surprising to find that the annual council sheltered housing total went from 14,375 to 36, but in the same period the housing association total also dropped, from 2425 to 838. This sharp drop in specialized new provision came in a period when more disabled people were living in the community and when the number of older people was growing. Over the same period of time, of course, 'ordinary' house-building in the public sector was decimated. It is difficult to envisage how different the options for older people might have been if building had continued, and had kept pace with changing standards and expectations.

In bricks and mortar, then, as in the issue of housework and other support services, provision shrank just as it particularly needed to expand. In her report, *A Life Worth Living*, Tessa Harding (1997) brought together the views of older people and the statistical information which showed the extent to which people in all tenures were being failed at every level by the systems that prevailed – with fewer options and ever less autonomy.

6

Maintaining independence: repair, adaptations and design

Provided housing is acceptably located and securely occupied, there are three main aspects which are necessary to help older people maintain independence. One is a home that is sufficiently warm, economical to run and in fit condition so it does not make the occupants ill with either pneumonia or anxiety; the second is help available when needed with housework, decorating, odd jobs and gardening; the third is design or adaptation that allows access to all the rooms and facilities of the home for those who can no longer walk, climb or bend as well as they once could.

The reduction or elimination of housework services to older people in the 1990s was a major impediment to successful independent living. However, the same period saw some really forward thinking and constructive developments of value to older people in the field of renovation, adaptation and new build, and these form the main subject of this chapter.

The problems of disrepair from an older person's viewpoint

The longer anyone of any age has lived in the same property, the more likely it is to be in poor condition (Leather 1993: 32). A person is most likely to look actively for defects in a property at the time when they are deciding whether or not to move in – and faults are most clearly visible when a house is stripped of furniture and fittings. If someone is buying, the surveyor will point out problems and the mortgage lender may require action as a condition of the loan. If you are a prospective tenant, with little chance of another move once you accept an offer, you are again likely to look with a critical eye and negotiate hard with the landlord about repairs. It is easiest, too, to decorate a property before moving in (and decorating often leads to minor repairs) and it is natural to do so to establish a sense of 'ownership'.

Once someone has moved in, however, the task will be harder and the motivation less. After a while, people get used to the defects of the home. Researchers talking to older people about their view of the physical state of their homes found that some 'tolerate . . . the house like an eccentric relative, not expecting great things from something of such an age' (Gurney and Means 1993: 124).

Older people simply because they are older and because they move less frequently (as Chapter 5 described) are likely to have lived longer in their homes and are particularly subject to the processes described above. The English House Condition Surveys (EHCS) that are carried out every five years have consistently found a correlation between levels of unfitness and the age of the occupants (see for example DoE 1993). The proportion of unfit dwellings among all households in England was 7.4 per cent in the 1991 survey.[1] In the age group 65–74, the figure was 6.9 per cent: lower than the average but higher than for the age groups between 35 and 54. In households headed by someone aged 75–84, however, the proportion of unfit housing was 10.3 per cent; and for those over 85 it was 13.3 per cent. Only among very young households were similar levels to be found (12.5 per cent for those aged 16–24) (Leather 1999: 55). The reasons for these figures are the subject of much debate, but one factor that the very old and the very young had in common in 1991 was that they were more likely than the rest of the population to be living in private rented accommodation; 36.9 per cent of households headed by someone over 75 in private rented accommodation in England in 1991 were found to be living in housing unfit for human habitation as legally defined (Leather 1999: 55). Another factor uniting the youngest and oldest adults is low income.

Tolerance not be confused with indifference

The fact that people over 75 are more likely to live in poor conditions and to accept them should not be confused with either ignorance or indifference to problems of disrepair. What should be understood is that, in addition to the tendencies to neglect that come from being in the same place a long time, which are not age specific, come some additional problems. People can perhaps no longer safely climb ladders (dizziness and poor balance are extremely common in later life). This means there will be a growing number of jobs they cannot do for themselves. At the same time, with a reduced income, it is harder to pay market prices for repairs or decoration and there is considerable well-based anxiety about finding a trustworthy builder. This may become more daunting still when those you have used for many years themselves retire or die. There is also the 'is it worth it?' factor. This relates both to the disruption of having builders in and the expense that will not be reflected in increased market value of the property. If someone expects to live only another two or three years, they may feel it is a waste of money repairing their home and they would rather have the cash available for themselves or to leave to their children.

Tolerance borne of long residence; inability to undertake work directly; high costs of employing others; fear of disruption and fear of exploitation and a feeling that the expense may prove a waste of money – these are all key factors in understanding why the 83-year-old living in that rather shabby property next door does not rush to do it up.

There is a school of thought that older people and others who neglect their properties, mainly those on low incomes, often do not know that their homes are in poor condition and that information (education) is therefore part of the solution. It is an orthodoxy based chiefly on the fact that, in housing satisfaction surveys, people in very poor condition houses have said they are satisfied with their homes, or even been so specific as to say the condition of their home is satisfactory, when objective judgement by surveyors shows it to be very poor. However, as Chapter 5 noted, other research (for example Heywood 1997) shows that the problem has lain in the wording of housing satisfaction questionnaires, which have asked people to cover too much in one answer. If older people are given the opportunity to differentiate between the objective state of their home and their emotional feelings about it, they are well aware when the roof is leaking, the walls damp and the windows draughty and ill fitting.

Older people may have a number of other reasons for not readily admitting problems with their housing. They may dread the disruption and cost of putting a problem right; they may feel they would not be able to find a trustworthy builder. Or, depending on where they live, they may feel that if they draw attention to their living conditions, they could be faced with compulsory purchase and clearance, or with strong pressure to move. Tenants of private landlords may further feel that complaint may lead to harassment, or improvement to rent rises (Smith 1989).

Taken together, these factors may help to create an impression of indifference to poor housing conditions, but where such factors have been understood, apparent indifference can turn into a strong desire for improvement.

Home improvement agencies

Origins

More commonly known as Staying Put or Care and Repair, these voluntary home improvement agencies began to develop in the early 1980s. This was part of the general trend, in the face of economic constraints, to renovation as an alternative to new build. There were long waiting lists for sheltered housing but the generous supply of housing association grant to build it was drying up. There were also people who did not relish sheltered housing and wanted to stay in their homes (Smith 1989). Finding a way to help some older people improve their living conditions without the need to move was one solution, and it was housing associations, notably Anchor, who pioneered and funded the early schemes. In the Local Government and Housing Act 1989, home improvement agencies received official government endorsement and some revenue funding was made available in England from the Department of the Environment (now DETR) and, in Wales, the Welsh Office (now the Welsh National Assembly). In the 1990s, as circumstances changed again, some agencies began to offer 'move on' services as a supplement to the 'staying put' option.

In the year 2000 there were 220 home improvement agencies in England,[2] and 26 in Wales,[3] besides some additional in-house agencies run by local authorities. In England, 86 per cent of agencies received DETR subsidy (Care and Repair England 1999: 12). In Wales, all the 26 agencies received funding from the Welsh Assembly, from the relevant local authority and from a parent housing association or group of housing associations. One-fifth were also receiving funding from their local health authority, in connection with projects for accident prevention or discharge from hospital. There was also some charitable funding, usually for short-term innovative projects. The system of direct funding to agencies from the DETR or Welsh Assembly, however, was due, at the time this book went to press, to be replaced under the *Supporting People* arrangements (DSS 1998b) with a block grant to agencies coming instead via the local authority out of its *Supporting People* budget.

How organized

Most home improvement agencies are extremely small. They employ usually just three or four workers: a coordinator/case worker who runs the agency and visits clients to discuss their needs, plan the work and raise funds, a technical officer who arranges and supervises the building work, and an administrator. If there is an extra staff member, it is likely to be an extra case worker, as advocacy is the core business of a home improvement agency. The idea is that the HIA case workers who visit an older person will listen carefully to their needs and respect their wishes. When only a small job is requested – even if the whole house is in need of repair – the HIA will not push the householder to have more. They will give time to listen and this is very much appreciated.[4]

An HIA offers whatever help is needed: filling in a grant application, drawing up plans or organizing tenders. The agency will offer a list of approved builders and supervise the work when in progress. If money needs to be found outside the grant system, they will do a benefits check and also pursue charities and other forms of funding where necessary. In short, the theory is that they lift the burdensome aspects of responsibility off the shoulders of the older person while not taking away the control: help rather than 'care' (Clark *et al.* 1998).

If agency clients have work done through a housing grant, the agency may charge a fee, which may be paid out of the individual's grant. These fees help towards running costs, but HIAs have no direct resources to pay for repair work. Sometimes local authorities will give an agency a notional share of the grants budget to which the agency's clients may apply, or give them responsibility for particular grants (with the authority merely giving approvals). In general, however, the agencies must use the systems that are available to all. This makes them advocates or conduits rather than benefactors, and is probably a great strength. Their added value is their expertise, local knowledge, reputation for trustworthiness and the quality of support they give to older people, who know that they can return to the agency if something goes wrong after work is completed, or if a new problem arises.

Good home improvement agencies are valuable to older people because, by design, they match the needs older people express, by offering direct practical help of the kind that is wanted to the degree that it is wanted. One client described how the local Care and Repair agency helped her to leave hospital by being willing to send someone to move her bed from upstairs to the ground floor when the statutory agencies had apparently no means of doing this.[5]

As these agencies have developed, some have taken on new tasks beyond their original remit. The large Care and Repair agency in Bristol has a quilting group, set up in response to the issue of loneliness that so many clients expressed. In contrast with lunch clubs or day centres, the quilting group requires a creative input from its members and has made a considerable impact on their lives, giving new purpose, new status and new friendships. Care and Repair Bristol has also joined Hackney Staying Put and a number of Welsh agencies in establishing a hospital discharge project. Other initiatives from Care and Repair agencies have included accident prevention, handy-person services and links with GP practices to help prevent admissions to hospital.

Main problems for HIAs

Because home improvement agencies are such small organizations, there will sometimes be projects which do not work well because of the failings of a single member of the team. In such circumstances, long waiting lists may be established and other professionals and clients alike may lose confidence in the ability of the agency to deliver. It is also very important that relationships between the HIA and local authority officers are good and their roles seen as complementary, not threatening.

The main problem for older people, however, is that for two out of three who need their services, no agency is available. They serve only certain areas, and within those areas only certain groups. They are not allowed by government to have more than 5 per cent of their clients from the social housing sector, and in most areas they help chiefly owners on incomes at or around benefit level. Many other owners would benefit from their support. An HIA with 3 members of staff can assist about 150 people a year, therefore 220 agencies are enough to serve about 33,000 people a year. We estimate that the number of agencies needs to go up to at least 600 if Help the Aged's objective of home improvement agencies to cover every area of the UK is to be achieved (Harding 1997: 17). At the moment, HIAs hardly dare to advertise for fear of creating demand they could not fulfil, so many who need their services are unaware of their existence.

Grants for renovation and repair

The Housing and Local Government Act 1989, which endorsed home improvement agencies and introduced some government-funded support for them, also introduced two new housing grants that were beneficial to older people whose homes were in disrepair. These were the mandatory renovation grant (which was abolished in 1996 and replaced with a discretionary grant) and minor works assistance (MWA), since 1996 renamed home repairs assistance (HRA).

Minor works/home repairs assistance

The minor works assistance grant was tailor made for older people, being a response to the knowledge coming out of the early home improvement agencies (Leather and Mackintosh 1992). It was a discretionary grant for people aged 60 and over, home-owners and all tenants in permanent dwellings except council tenants. Anyone in receipt of income support or other means-tested benefit was eligible for 100 per cent grant with no further means test and no need for a social services assessment (see below under disabled facilities grant). For those who needed work done to remain in their home, there was the version of minor works assistance called 'Staying Put grant', which could be used for repairs or adaptation. For those wishing to move there was the 'elderly person's adaptation grant', which could be used to adapt another person's home to make it suitable. The grant limit was £1080, but three grants could be given in a three-year period and some authorities contrived to give two or even three in close succession in order to be able to use them for bigger jobs such as re-roofing.

From its inception to its replacement by home repairs assistance in 1996, the value of an average minor works assistance grant was around £650 (Heywood and Smart 1996: 50), though this figure conceals the cases where multiple grant was used. Minor works assistance was ideal for older people because it could be given quickly with a minimum of fuss and bureaucracy and be used (within the funding limit) for exactly what the older person wanted, however small. There was no requirement that the whole house be made fit, as there was with renovation and disabled facilities grants, so frail older people who did not want the upheaval of major repairs could be helped to have just a door replaced, a new boiler, some replacement windows or whatever the pressing problem was. The provision for further applications also made it possible for second thoughts to be had if the first work was a success.

Home improvement agencies were particularly well placed to make use of minor works assistance and some local authorities allocated all or some of their minor works assistance budgets to these agencies to use at their discretion. Agencies could claim a percentage of the grant (8 or 10 per cent was common) as a fee for their work, but with small grants such a fee was very unlikely to cover the costs involved. Moreover, when more expensive work was needed the agencies sometimes waived the fee in order to leave the full amount of grant available to the applicant. These two factors meant that although minor works assistance (subsequently home repairs assistance) was very important to the work that agencies were able to do, fees from them did not bring in significant funding to help the agencies stay in existence.

Minor works assistance was popular with older people, with agencies and with local authorities. The major disadvantage of it, and of home repairs assistance, was that it was discretionary, and local authorities were forced by lack of funds to contain the numbers given regardless of demand. In England expenditure rose only from £18 million to £20.4 million between 1991–2 and 1994–5, and in Wales in the same period it actually went down from £5 million to £3.5 million. The problem between 1990 and 1996 was the huge demand for mandatory grants (renovation and disabled facilities) which made some authorities decide they could give no discretionary grants, despite knowing the usefulness of minor works assistance. When, however, the mandatory renovation grant was abolished, in 1996, local authorities were free to choose to give either home repairs assistance or renovation grant, as they pleased. With shrinking budgets, they were naturally more inclined to help more people with smaller grants. In these circumstances, the number of minor works or home repairs assistance grants, completed in England, which had remained at about 30,000 a year from 1994 to 1997, rose steeply in 1998 and 1999, to 50,375 and 65,024 respectively. Because of the higher ceiling, in the same period the average cost also rose from around £700 to around £1000 and total expenditure went from £24 million in 1996 to £63 million in 1999, with similar increases in Wales (DETR 1999b: Table 7.3; DETR 2000b: Table 2.18).

Home repairs assistance in the year 2000

At the time of writing, home repairs assistance may be given to anyone of any age who is in receipt of a means-tested benefit, but also to any person over 60, regardless of income. The advantages described above relating to minor works assistance still apply to home repairs assistance: it is quick, non-bureaucratic, flexible and efficient. Terms in 2000 were one home repairs assistance grant of up to £2000 or two in a three-year period to a maximum of £4000.

Mandatory renovation grant: its rise, fall and significance to older people

The mandatory renovation grant introduced in the Local Government and Housing Act 1989 and abolished in 1996 represented an endeavour to end the problem of unfit housing in England and Wales. Through its provisions, anyone owning or living in a privately owned property more than ten years old which was 'unfit for human habitation' as then legally defined was entitled to a grant to make it 'fit'. A Test of Resources (means test) laid down by government was applied to ensure that anyone applying must first contribute the maximum their income would allow. The essential points were that it was based on housing benefit rules and took only income, not outgoings, into account. Most specifically it made no recognition of real mortgage costs, allowing only a figure (£40 per week) which was about half the average national mortgage cost in 1996. Some older people (those on low incomes who owned their homes outright) benefited from this system, though it heavily penalized those who had higher incomes but who also had mortgages or other debts. Despite the tight restrictions, however, demand from people of all ages who were sufficiently poor to qualify was huge and was not matched with increased resources. Local authorities pleaded to government that they could not cope and in 1996 the Housing Grants, Construction and Regeneration Act removed the link between an 'unfit' home and the right to a grant, and returned full discretion in the giving of renovation grants to local housing authorities.

This period of mandatory renovation grant linked to unfitness, although it is now over, is mentioned because it was in force just long enough to show how much such a system is needed for older people, and how it gave help to those who had formerly been excluded and who are now excluded once more. Local authorities in areas with a lot of poor housing prefer to concentrate their efforts in particular areas, rather than 'pepper-potting' (that is spreading their resources so thinly there is no discernible improvement). In the period between 1990 (when the 1989 Act took effect) and 1996, however, authorities could not legally confine applications to such areas.

In 1992–3, researchers in Birmingham interviewed a range of people who had applied (some successfully, some not) for grants under the new legislation, to discover their views of the system.[6] These researchers were familiar with the housing problems of Birmingham's inner areas and supportive of the city's area-focused policies, but the project brought them into contact with new and hidden needs: mostly very serious and mainly affecting older people. There were owner-occupiers in middle-income districts whose incomes had been drastically reduced by widowhood, illness or redundancy; there were people in scattered blocks of old terraced housing or isolated older properties in mainly newer-built areas, and people in inter-war or post-1945 housing also in grave need of repair. Most of the older people in the sample had qualified for grant aid because their incomes were so low and their housing was unfit. They had received help because the local authority at this time could no longer confine grant aid to specific geographical areas as they had preferred to do before. These older owners described the misery they had suffered before the relief of having at last had help, and the peace of mind it gave them to know the roof had been repaired and deterioration of the property halted. 'In the past I've had the roof patched and patched. I can sleep at night now'. 'I've been here 58 years. It needed rewiring – it had never been done in that time and I was really worried – I went to Age Concern'. 'There's plenty of old people in houses built in the 1930s who can't afford to do anything. Their houses are deteriorating. Publicity for grants bypasses those who need help'.

These quotations illustrate the kinds of housing needs that mandatory renovation grant, while it existed, both uncovered and remedied. Home repairs assistance is not sufficient to meet the costs of these more serious problems.

Non-mandatory renovation grants

After the passing of the Housing Grants, Construction and Regeneration Act 1996 there was no longer any mandatory right to renovation grant. In the year 2000 an older owner wanting help to convert or renovate a property could still ask their local housing authority about a renovation grant, but with only a small chance of obtaining it because budgets had been so much reduced. The details of items for which such grants might be given were spelt out in the Act at section 27 (DoE 1997: 16). They included not only remedying unfitness as legally defined, but also providing insulation, improving heating facilities, providing fire escapes or precautions and providing 'satisfactory internal arrangement'. Renovation grants could also be given to help convert a non-dwelling into a dwelling, or a single family dwelling into flats.

Where renovation grants are given, they commonly include such things as repairing or replacing roofs, gutters, windows and doors; replacing unsafe gas and water pipes and broken drains; rewiring; installing a damp-proof course; installing a bathroom or inside toilet; improving ventilation and dealing with problems of rot, besides the items listed above relating to arrangement, heating, insulation and escape from fire. It is possible, however, to have a renovation grant which remedies unfitness and does not greatly improve the comfort of living in a property, especially if only minimal work is done to the kitchen, central heating is not installed and bad old plasterwork inside is patched up rather than replaced. The grant must leave the property 'fit' – but the result can leave a property looking very knocked about and be disappointing for the occupant, depending on the authority's policies on standards. Home improvement agencies which are able to arrange decoration following renovation may make all the difference.

To ensure that the grant system helped people who genuinely wanted better living conditions but was not abused by profiteers, the 1996 Act imposed conditions. Renovation grants could be given only to those who had lived at least three years in a property, and had to be repaid (on a sliding scale) if the property were sold within five years after the grant was given. But we need to acknowledge in this chapter that in the case of home improvement, legislators have understood the needs of older people. In general terms, the secretary of state was given authority to vary these conditions nationally, and local authorities could also waive them locally, but for the needs of older people the Act was more directly specific and helpful. At paragraph 45 of Part 1, Chapter 1 of the Act, it states that repayment of grant at the point of a sale within five years does *not* apply in cases where the owner of the dwelling is elderly or infirm and is making the disposal with the intention

> of going to live in a hospital, hospice, sheltered housing, residential care home or similar institution as his only or main residence,
>
> or
>
> of moving to somewhere where care will be provided by any person.
>
> (DoE 1997: 28)

This provision means that not only do older people who move for valid reasons within five years not have to repay the grant, but also they can be reassured on this point if they express anxiety as to whether it is worth having the work done at all.

Similar reassurance may be given to grant applicants who are not old themselves but know they may have to move at some time in order to care for a parent or other family members. The Act excludes from the obligation of repayment any owner who '(b) is making the disposal with the intention of going to live with and care for an elderly or infirm member of his family or his partner's family' (DoE 1997: 28).

Changes proposed to the grant system in early twenty-first century

In 1998, a consultation paper on the fitness standard (DETR 1998b) proposed changes which, at the time of writing, were expected to be consolidated in new legislation. It is extremely likely that more items, including thermal efficiency, internal arrangement, fire safety and radon gas will be taken into account in assessing fitness. A graduated fitness rating is expected to replace or supplement the pass or fail fitness standard, and more account will be taken of the likely effects on the occupants of anything that is defective. This approach will be less housing-stock focused than the system it will replace and may eventually alter the perspectives of the professionals engaged in renewal. These changes could be beneficial to older people whose housing is putting their health at risk, providing the change in legislation is backed with resources for action.

Other likely changes were contained in the Housing Green Paper (DETR 2000a). These, however, were not very encouraging. The subject of the nation's unfit owner-occupied housing merited just 2 pages of the 130 page report. The proposals were to give to local authorities either increased or absolute discretion in the giving of grants (except for disabled facilities grants), to offer loans as an alternative to grants, and to hope that money to improve poor condition privately owned housing could be found through equity release or private finance. The word 'discretion' should sound alarm bells. The proposals suggest that for the moment the government was hoping the problem of poor condition housing would solve itself through the market, although the history of the past hundred years suggests that this is highly unlikely. Meanwhile the implications for older people needing financial help with the cost of repairs looked likely to be bad because of the lack of funding. Budgets for private sector renewal in England went down from £303 million to £165 million between 1993 and 1999 (DETR 1999b: 6). From 2000 onwards there will be no specified budget for renewal and funding will have to be sought in the bidding process at local authority level.

Other sources of financial help with home improvement

From time to time, new or short-term projects designed to help improve housing conditions are put forward. In 1998, for example, the Department of Health's (1998a) White Paper, *Modernising Social Services*, announced a 'Prevention Grant' totalling £100 million over three years to stimulate local authorities into developing strategies beginning in 2000 to 'prevent or delay loss of independence', with older people as the main intended beneficiaries. Among the examples of preventive strategies given in the White Paper were 'home safety checks and handyperson schemes' and 'providing speedier access to equipment and adaptation'. The guidance to this White Paper stipulates that, as a condition of grant, social services authorities have to show how they will agree a three-year plan with health authorities and how they have worked in partnership with other organizations, *'especially housing departments in drawing up the strategy'* (DoH 1998a, added emphasis). Evidence from Care and Repair Cymru suggests that by 2000 similar policies in Wales were already having a noticeable effect, with support coming from social services authorities for a growth in accident prevention and handyperson schemes.

In 1999, too, the government announced a new phase of the longstanding Home Energy Efficiency Scheme (HEES) which had, in fits and starts, offered some help with insulation and draught proofing to people on low incomes. 'New HEES' contained a provision exclusive to people over 60 in receipt of a means-tested benefit for a higher grant (up to £2000) and permission to use it for the installation of a partial central heating system, not just for insulation.

Adaptations for older people: the move towards social inclusion

Very few older people use the term 'disabled' of themselves. Chapter 2 in the discussion of the social model of disability noted that the concept has not yet achieved widespread use among older people. However, because the idea of the social model of disability has been so important and influential in achieving change at the end of the twentieth century, throughout this section we bear it in mind.

Many older people are disabled by their own housing and socially excluded by that of their friends and relatives. Chapter 5 explored the many ways domestic environments make life hard for older people. These problems can be removed by alterations to housing, commonly referred to as 'adaptations'. The nature and extent of such provision says much about society's attitude towards older people. In tracing briefly the development of state help with adaptations, and the debates about how they should be funded, we shall therefore also be tracing the models of disability and old age that have underpinned the policies.

Chronically Sick and Disabled Persons Act 1970

The rights of older people to have adaptations to their homes were first clearly stated in the Chronically Sick and Disabled Persons (CSDP) Act 1970. Although it has been tarnished and dented by the Gloucestershire judgment of 1997,[7] the Act is still in 2000 a powerful declaration of the duties of society towards those who are impaired in any way, mentally or physically and those who are chronically sick. However, it is based on a view of disability which critics have described as 'one of individualised social limitations' (Stewart *et al.* 1999: 5).

Part 1 of the CSDP Act gave to the relevant local authorities (in effect, any social services authority) a duty to discover the numbers of people to whom section 29 of the National Assistance Act 1948 applied (section 1); a duty to publish general information about the services they provided to people as defined in Section 29 (section 2(a)); and a duty to inform any one receiving any one of those services, of any other service relevant to their needs (section 2(b)).[8] All these duties were still applicable in the year 2000.

Part 2 listed the welfare provision that local authorities had a duty to make arrangements to provide if they were necessary to meet the needs of the disabled person. This list of items (a) to (h) includes 'practical assistance' in the home and '(e) the provision of assistance for that person in arranging for the carrying out of any works of adaptation in his home or the provision of any additional facilities designed to secure his greater safety, comfort or convenience' (DoH 1970: section 2(e)).

From 1970 onwards, therefore, a duty to provide adaptations to the homes of disabled people lay with social services authorities. They employed occupational therapists to assess the needs, specify the work, and often (if it was a matter of fitting a grab rail) even carry it out themselves. The majority of clients needing this service were older people. What was done was fairly basic (ramps, grab rails, handrails) and there was normally no charge the work was paid for by social services or (in the case of council tenants and the tiny number of housing association tenants) the landlord. For more complex work (widening doors, fitting showers and lifts) social services often employed their own team of technicians, as some still do.

Local Government and Housing Act 1989

Between 1970 and 1989, the need for adaptations changed in quality, quantity and cost. More seriously disabled people wanted to live in homes of their own – and to do so they needed more expensive and extensive adaptations, including, often, an extension to house a downstairs bathroom or bedroom. More sophisticated equipment also became available. These changes coincided with the moves described above towards renovation rather than redevelopment. Social services authorities found that instead of paying the full costs of these more expensive adaptations, they could encourage the use of housing renovation grants for the purpose and pay only the owner's contribution to grant of 25 or 10 per cent. The growing use of improvement grants for adaptation coincided with the growth of the early home improvement agencies; consequential knowledge and understanding of older people's repair and adaptation needs and the continued move in society against residential institutions. Matters were regularized in the Local Government and Housing Act 1989. For disabled people this was another landmark in terms of civil rights, although from the government perspective it was more to do with their general agenda of reducing the cost to government of residential care. 'The adaptation, where necessary, of existing dwellings occupied by elderly and disabled people is often a pre-requisite for the success of community care' (NHS and Community Care Act 1990: section 7).

The 1989 Act introduced, for the first time, not only a general right to have adaptation provided by welfare professionals but also a mandatory disabled facilities grant, with detailed provisions. Specified items included access in and out of the property, access to bathroom, toilet, own bedroom, living room and kitchen, suitable heating, access to light, power and heating switches and access to other rooms if the disabled or older person needed this to care for someone else. Maximum amounts were identical to those for renovation grant: unlimited when the Act was passed, but reduced to a maximum of £20,000 (£24,000 in Wales) from April 1994 onwards. The Test of Resources was also basically the same as for renovation grant, with the same adverse effects.

Symbolically, the introduction of this mandatory disabled facilities grant was important. To some extent, it made adaptation a matter of housing rights shared by all people rather than of welfare provision for a group in need of care. But there was still the requirement that the welfare authority must recommend that the adaptations were 'necessary and appropriate', so the model was not essentially a social one, but only a step in that direction. It set out to remove the barriers that disabled people encountered in their homes and its provisions mirrored the rights to 'fit' housing set out in the same Act in the provisions for renovation grant. People without a bath or proper kitchen were entitled to have one; people who could not gain access to their bath or kitchen were similarly entitled. The 1989 Act made no distinctions on grounds of age. The foreword of the joint circular that was issued by the Department of the Environment and the Department of Health in 1990 strongly emphasizes the humanity and individuality of applicants, the need to consider psychological factors and the need to consult with the grant applicants (DoE/DoH 1990: sections 27, 28, 38).

The 1989 Act fails older people

In practice, however, there were major problems with the 1989 adaptation provisions (Heywood 1996: 126–38). The effectiveness of the new mandatory grant was marred by the Test of Resources, by the shortage of assessment staff, by the lack of social services policies and capital to help applicants who could not afford their contributions and by shortage of a capital and revenue funding in grants departments. Certain key issues affected older people in particular. The Test of Resources was applied not only to the disabled person and their spouse but also to the owner of the property, hitting families where an older person needing adaptations was living with a grown-up child (a form of institutional discrimination against extended families). The Test of Resources itself was based on the principle that help would be given only after the applicant had put in the maximum they could afford to borrow, according to a government formula. This penalized older people with small occupational pensions, who were likely to get no help at all. It also hurt those who, perhaps because they were old enough to remember the humiliation of the Poor Law means test, refused to go through it at all. There was a requirement, too, that the property be made 'fit' before adaptation, which not only caused delay in achieving the needed adaptation but also meant major upheaval for some older people. Delay itself was perhaps the biggest problem of all. The Act required an assessment by 'the welfare authority' before a grant could be given. The growth in demand, shortage of capital and a widespread shortage of the community occupational therapists who were qualified to make these assessments meant that the Social Services Inspectorate found 'a disturbing picture with the average wait of 11 months [for a first assessment] being quite unsatisfactory' (Social Services Inspectorate 1994: 10).

Discrimination against older people

The result of long waiting lists for assessment in some areas was prioritizing by the social services authority, and in this process older people lost out very badly indeed. One southern authority policy paper put all older people into priority 3, 'other', and said that people in this category would not generally receive any service. Others tried to stem the demand for adaptation assessment visits by excluding in advance older people who wanted 'only' bathing adaptations or 'only' central heating (see Chapter 3 for discussion of the community care charter; see also Heywood and Smart 1996: 101). These decisions were made not because managers necessarily believed bathing and heating to be unimportant, but precisely because they were so important to so many people that demand was exceedingly high, and a real dent in the waiting lists would be made if they were declared ineligible.

These actions disbarring older people from their mandatory rights illustrate another structural problem with the 1989 Act. Despite the issuing of a joint circular by the Department of Health and the Department of the Environment (DoE/DoH 1990), the legislation was in a Housing Act and was either misunderstood or ignored by too many senior managers in social services departments. So much did some misunderstand it that they dispensed completely with a budget for adaptations because they thought all the costs would henceforth be borne by housing. This indicates that they had not acknowledged that the Test of Resources for disabled facilities grants would exclude many applicants and that the cumbersome disabled facilities grant process was not suitable for minor adaptations (of which thousands are given every year in every authority). There was also apparent unawareness of the continuing duty of social services to fulfil its obligations under the CSDP Act 1970 whenever the housing grant system could not help. Once again, older people lost out because the effects of poor service to them were private and hidden. Change in this arena became a national issue only when the wait for adaptation assessments became the most common cause of complaint to the local government Ombudsman. Before that, local occupational therapy managers had to do whatever they could locally to try to ease the situation.

The net impact of the introduction of disabled facilities grant in the first four years was that the total amount of housing grant money being spent on adaptations in England went down not up. In 1990 national grant on adaptations spending completed under the old legislation had been £68.8 million. This dropped to £50.2 million in 1991 and was still only £61.4 million in 1993. Social services expenditure on adaptations also went down from £24.5 million to £21 million between 1990 and 1991, for reasons already discussed, rising to £26 million in 1992 and 1993 (Heywood and Smart 1996: 88).

The figures are all the more strange since it is estimated that requests for adaptations increased by an average of 50 per cent nationally during the same years (1991–4) that grant funding was going down. By contrast, in this same period, the amount spent by the Housing Corporation on adaptations more than doubled (from £5.4 million to £11.8 million) while the amount spent by hard-pressed local authority housing departments also nearly doubled (from £45.3 million to £86 million), as they responded to the growth in demand. This received little attention, and the common understanding by all except those most closely involved was that disabled facilities grant had transformed the position of disabled and older people. As the figures show, this was not the case. The introduction of the disabled facilities grant was therefore at first a very effective illusory trick – appearing to give help while in fact, through its small print, it made help harder to get. The provisions of the grant themselves were, in theory, generous, but they were hedged about with bureaucratic provisions which left applicants as much as ever at the mercy of welfare 'assessment'.

Housing Grants, Construction and Regeneration Act 1996

This is the legislation that was current at the time of writing in 2000. It was one of three housing Acts put through Parliament in the fourth term of the then Conservative government, and its main and urgent purpose was to abolish mandatory renovation grants. It is extremely likely that the government would have liked at the same time to abolish mandatory disabled facilities grant. At this time, however, the disability movement had become very militant and active and had a lot of support in the press, so abolition of a right was probably judged inexpedient politically. In fact, organizations of and for disabled and older people were very active during the passage of this 1996 Act and secured a definition of 'disabled' that was unique to this Act (DoE 1997: section 100(1)).

Another major change in the 1996 Act was the provision that the Test of Resources was now to be applied only to the applicant and partner, not to others with an interest in the property. This meant that an older person living with an adult child could apply for disabled facilities grant without their child being penalized. In addition, the requirement to 'make fit' was removed, and a new clause relating to safety introduced. This could be used for enhanced lighting or enhanced alarms for anyone with poor eyesight or hearing, as well as more obvious safety measures.

The situation in 2000, therefore, was that an older person with any kind of problem that required an adaptation to their home could apply for disabled facilities grant. People in all tenures could do this, and there was no 'length of residence' qualification as there was for renovation grants. In two-tier authorities a social services occupational therapist from the county would first visit and decide whether an adaptation was necessary and appropriate and a housing authority officer would decide whether it was reasonable and practicable bearing in mind the age and condition of the property. In unitary authorities, the housing department could act on its own or employ health authority or even directly employed assessors, though most still worked through social services. The Test of Resources would be applied. Applicants who could not afford their contribution would be entitled to help from social services. The maximum mandatory grant (to be on top of whatever the applicant contributed) was £20,000 in England and £24,000 in Wales. The items for which grant *must* be given were the same as in the 1989 Act except for the extra provision of making the dwelling safe (DoE 1997: para 23(1)). In addition to the mandatory grant, there was a discretionary disabled facilities grant which could be given to an unlimited amount either to help pay for mandatory items if mandatory grant was insufficient or 'for making the dwelling or building suitable for the accommodation, welfare or employment of the disabled occupant in any other respect' (DoE 1997: section 23(2)).

The mandatory provisions about bathing and the lavatory were spelt out in even more detail than in the 1989 Act. This was because so many (mainly older) people were being refused bathing adaptations (and some were being offered a commode instead of an accessible toilet) that it was felt necessary to make the intentions of the legislation absolutely clear.

However, evidence collected by Age Concern and the Royal Association for Disability and Rehabilitation (RADAR) showed how some social services authorities were still saying that people must manage with a strip wash at the sink or a weekly bath at a day centre, and that if they had these things they did not qualify for an assessment (so were effectively disbarred from disabled facilities grant). 'Bathing is a low priority – clients can and have waited 18–24 months'. 'They [occupational therapists] . . . will not visit people at all if people can strip wash' (Age Concern and RADAR 1999: 4).

Tenure discrimination

For disabled facilities grants given in all tenures except council housing, local authorities at the time of writing received a 60 per cent subsidy from central government. The absence of this subsidy for council tenants meant there was no incentive for councils to offer full disabled facilities grant rights to their tenants. In 11 per cent of local authority areas, tenants who were 'under-occupying' were not offered adaptations, despite their legal entitlement, but asked to move to alternative council housing (Age Concern and RADAR 1999: 2–3). Other authorities put a maximum cash limit well below £20,000 on adaptations for their tenants, for the understandable reason that such investment would not lead to a corresponding increase in value of the stock. While the option of being able to move is desirable, and will be welcomed by some older people, everything that is known about the meaning of home and the need to avoid inducing feelings of helplessness suggests that these policies may be harmful to older people if they are forced to move rather than being offered a choice. Central government bears the prime responsibility for this discrimination.

What adaptations achieve for older people

The great majority of adaptations put in for older people are extremely simple: a grab rail by the front door step, a couple more by the bath and toilet and a second banister rail up the stairs. These things are cheap and unobtrusive, and what they give is 'that little bit of help' – just enough to make the difference between confidence and anxiety. Research ongoing at the time of writing

(Heywood 2001) gave an overwhelming endorsement of the benefits of these minor adaptations, with increased feelings of safety, ability to take a bath or shower, being more able to run the home and to go out and needing less help from others. Over three-quarters of those consulted said there had been a positively good effect on their health, and there were virtually no problems and no perceived waste.

Those consulted in the same study about more major alterations – extensions, stair-lifts, bathing adaptations – were also hugely positive about the transformation that good adaptations had brought to their quality of life. 'The shower put in in 1994 has been a Godsend. They made a good job of it and I do not know how I would manage without it'. 'The stair-lift has been an absolute Godsend. What used to take 15 mins now takes 1'. 'The effect of the intercom was also wonderful. Such a safe feeling not to have to open the door unless you know who is there. Every elderly person should have one'. 'Before the adaptations I was suffering terrible loss of dignity, loss of independence. For me this was terrible: always waiting on other people: "Could you go up and get me a cardigan?" Also, I hated being seen naked. I truly believe I wouldn't be alive without the adaptations – for psychological rather than physical reasons.'

One older woman in a large family stressed how she valued being able to care for the family again. Other benefits repeatedly listed in this research included reduction of pain and discomfort, reducing the struggle involved in personal tasks so as to leave more time and strength for enjoying life, making it possible to go out after being housebound, making it possible for people to feel independent again, and giving people back their self-respect and dignity. People's embarrassment and misery at having to have commodes in their living rooms or kitchens cannot be overstated.

The effectiveness of minor adaptations is such that it is clearly desirable to have separate, swift means of supplying these, as many good authorities do, and not categorize them as low priorities involving two-year waits. The distress, discomfort and risk suffered by people waiting for or denied major adaptations also needs to be taken on board and tackled. In some areas and some tenures there are no waiting lists for assessment, no prioritizing and no problems in funding what is needed (Age Concern England and RADAR 1999: 5). This could and should be the normal situation.

Adaptations and hospital discharge

It is estimated that in the late twentieth century there were annually about 100,000 emergency readmissions to hospital within 28 days of discharge of people over 75 (Harding 1997: 6). Evidence from older people consulted on this topic suggests that discharge before people are well enough, the abolition of convalescence (now reinvented as rehabilitation) and lack of care and support in the early days after discharge may well be contributory factors.

There are also people who are unable to go home, even when they are well enough, because of the complete unsuitability of their home and the need for adaptations before they can live there. The Department of Health workbook on hospital discharge raised this issue. 'Have any aids and adaptations which are required been supplied and fitted where necessary, and the patient and carer trained in their use?' (DoH 1994b: paragraph 41).

This question, however, seems very remote from the pressures on hospital staff to release beds and the length of time it takes to fund and organize adaptations. What is of grave concern is that in these circumstances vulnerable older people may be discharged into a nursing or residential home and never even be told of the option of having their home adapted.

Hospital discharge is an area where the need for close working between health, housing and social services is absolutely critical. Although some places have established good and fruitful cooperation, Clark *et al.* (1996) in their study of hospital discharge, showed the tensions and non-communication in one area between hospital occupational therapists and their counterparts working for social services and how these tensions worked against the interests of older people.

Lifetime Homes: the ultimate preventive measure

If all housing were built without steps to the outside doors, on one level only on each floor, with wide doors and passages, plenty of turning space for a wheelchair and a downstairs toilet big enough for a wheelchair to get in and to fit a shower if necessary, many adaptations would not be needed. If, in addition, houses of more than one storey had stairs designed so that it was easy to fit a stair-lift, and floors and ceilings suitable for fitting a through floor lift or tracking hoists, these items could be fitted with maximum ease and minimum expense if ever they were needed. If, finally, the inside were conceived with an older person in mind, including power sockets at waist height and windows low enough for a pleasant view from an armchair or wheelchair, the house or flat could be so much more convenient, without any need for alteration or extra expense later. This is the basic concept of the Lifetime Home, promoted by the Joseph Rowntree Foundation from 1991 onwards. The term implies a home which will suit a person throughout their lifetime, so that they are not forced to move by barriers in the dwelling. The level access and wide doors will benefit the parent with a double-buggy as well as a wheelchair user. Everyone will benefit from the slightly improved space standards.

In 1998, following a long campaign and promises given while the Labour Party were in opposition, the government introduced measures extending Part M of the building regulations (which specify provision for disabled people in public buildings) to all new-built domestic dwellings, in all tenures. From this time on, every new house and flat had to have a level or ramped approach, at least 900 mm wide; an accessible threshold; an entrance door with minimum 775 mm opening; a toilet at the entrance storey level usable by wheelchair users; corridors wide enough for wheelchair circulation; no changes of level on the entrance storey (except on steeply sloping sites) and switches and sockets between 450 mm and 1200 mm from the floor (DETR 1998c).

There were a few exceptions, and there are bound to be problems of enforcement. Builders and developers were hostile because the requirements would increase the costs of small houses. This legislation is, however, likely to be extremely beneficial to many people as they become older, not just as occupants but as visitors to other people's houses.

Assistive technology

The last decades of the twentieth century saw the development of a range of technological appliances relative to housing, some of which, like the door intercom mentioned above as an adaptation, have great potential for benefiting older people.

Early, widely used forms of assistive technology were external security lights, operated by movement- or light-sensitive sensors; smoke detectors; timed switches which would put on lights to deter burglars or switch on a cooker while the householder was out; alarms which could be used to summon help in case of an emergency; television and video remote controls, and, more recently, the ubiquitous mobile phone. For seriously disabled people there were also environmental control systems (ECS) that enabled someone to use remote control to open and close doors, draw curtains or operate other equipment, but in the 1980s and 1990s these were still very expensive. At the beginning of the twenty-first century, the range and ingenuity of assistive technology have expanded exponentially while its cost has come down, and there has been great interest in its potential to assist older people in their homes. There are devices which will sound an alarm in the event of a fall, even if the person who has fallen is not able to press a button. A sensor can be put on a door so that, if someone goes out at night or in the cold, a voice will tell them it is raining and remind them to put on a coat, and an alarm will sound if they have not come back through the door after a certain length of time. A gadget fixed to a door can take photographs of everyone who calls. If anyone living on the higher floors of a block of flats has a problem with remembering to turn off taps, technology can be arranged to detect the problem and switch off the water automatically.

When a number of possible devices are taken together and planned into a dwelling, the result is the 'Smart' house – the ultimate in designer living. A Smart house designed specifically with older people in mind has been developed in Gloucester and includes a locator device (press the picture on the wall and the lost item will beep), a bath monitor (checks level and temperature and tells you it is ready) and passive infrared sensors that detect the user's movements (Rickford 2000).

The issue of 'detecting the user's movements' serves as an indicator of the ethical issues surrounding the use of assistive technology. For whose benefit is it devised, and what model of human life, including old age, is it based in? The technology makes it possible for family or professionals to track every aspect of an older person's movements, including pulse rate, but how desirable is this?

Smith (1986) noted that by no means all older people welcomed even the presence of a warden and that 'the notion of alarm systems can evoke images of "Big Brother"' (Smith 1986: 15). If doubts were felt about alarms controlled by the individuals themselves, what will people feel about mechanisms that record every visit to the toilet (or fridge)?

Other ethical implications of assistive technology are taken up by Cowan and Turner-Smith (1999) on the subject for the Royal Commission on Long Term Care for the Elderly. Their concern is primarily that technology should be offered in a way that is psychologically acceptable to older people.

> Often, however, an important reason for rejection [of assistive technology] is the stigma attached to an assistive product. Services provide technology to meet a 'need', but users . . . will most readily use technology that is desirable because it enhances their social status as well as enabling them to do things or making them feel better . . . design for older people at home has to be based on want, not an assumption of need.
>
> (Royal Commission 1999, vol. 2: 335)

Cowan and Turner-Smith (1999) see that the danger lies in working from a medical model of old age or disability, that many older people 'may have difficulty in defining themselves as disabled or in need of special equipment' and that equipment, if it is to be used, must 'add ability without removing status' (Cowan and Turner-Smith 1999: 327). It is better, they suggest, to have items on the market that people of all ages will want, than to foist helpful 'disability' gadgets on to reluctant recipients.

Perhaps the key issue here is that, up to now, most assistive technology has been designed primarily for the benefit of professionals or family. Its function is to prevent them worrying and to ensure increased safety for the person themselves and for others, such as neighbours, who might be affected by a flood or fire, while reducing the number of actual visits necessary.

If older people themselves were being asked what kind of assistive technology they might like, would they want facilities which reduced human contact? And would they not perhaps ask for the means to clean windows and change curtains and light bulbs, do the housework or gardening, or be able to keep driving despite worsening eyesight. This is pure speculation, but is included to illustrate the general point that at present much of the new technology is 'assisting' other people, not older people themselves.

Broader design issues

Design issues for older people could go beyond even the provisions envisaged by Lifetime Homes. In Chapter 5 we considered the idea of designing specifically for older people options so attractive that younger people would be envious. While renovation and adaptation will both be necessary for many years to come, it makes social, economic and ecological sense to ensure that new dwellings are attractive, versatile and well built. Brenton's (1998) work on co-housing in the Netherlands shows a model worth considering, she particularly contrasts the spacious room sizes of the Dutch model (Brenton 1998). It must be remembered, however, that at any given time, most older people will be living in the houses they lived in when they were younger, not in specialized housing. The key to better housing for large numbers of older people therefore lies in better design, quality and space standards in all housing, public and private.

Conclusion

This chapter has been concerned with some of the practical bricks and mortar issues of housing for older people. Some in-depth discussion of policy developments has been provided to illustrate the complex intertwining of need, legislation, resources, implementation and the power and influence of particular models of ageing.

Within the housing legislation built up in the 1980s and 1990s, there were devised a great array of policy and practice tools appropriate for older householders: home repairs assistance, Home Energy Efficiency Schemes, renovation grant, disabled facilities grants, good regulations for new build, and home improvement agencies offering support even when funding is not a problem. Some of this legislation is quite powerful and not ageist. The fear of disruption, the unpredictability of old age and the need for support is well understood. In theory the grants available are varied, flexible and appropriate to a great range of needs. However, the reality is that there continues to be an enormous gulf between the need for good quality and appropriate housing and its supply. A severe lack of funding is, of course, the key problem, but there are others. The ineffectiveness of joint working (a subject we deal with in Chapter 8) continues to hamper the effective delivery services that improve homes. This chapter has shown that 'cost shunting' by different agencies bedevils the housing and community care system.

The final problem relates to attitude. Although the legislation may not be ageist, the people who deliver services are not always attuned to the principles behind the social model of disability. Policies for refusing services to older people are not made simply because of shortage of resources but arguably due to deep-seated attitudes relating to power and control reminiscent of the values of the Charity Organization Society discussed in Chapter 1.

Notes

1 By the time this book was going to press the 1996 EHCS was available. However, changes in the way data were presented for older people made it difficult for us to exploit and compare with previous surveys.
2 Private communication from Foundations, the national coordinating body for HIAs in England, August 2000.
3 Private communication with Care and Repair Cymru, August 2000.
4 From 1997 onwards Heywood has each year invited clients of Care and Repair Bristol to address students on a housing course. The views expressed by these clients have enriched the published sources (see for example Smith 1989; Mackintosh and Leather 1992) as a source of information.
5 Talk given at meeting of Age Concern Bristol and Brunel Care research forum, 19 January 2000.
6 This work led into Birmingham's Community Forum Submission, in 1993, to the DoE on the 1989 Act.
7 Regina v Gloucestershire County Counciland the Secretary of State for Health (Appellant) *ex parte* Barry (A.P.) (Respondent) 20 March 1997. The essence of the Law Lords' ruling in this case was that local authorities could take their own resources into account when assessing need, although they must not withdraw or reduce services without reassessing.

8 The definition of 'disabled' in the CSDP 1970 Act was taken from section 29 of the National Assistance Act 1948 'persons aged eighteen or over who are blind, deaf or dumb or who suffer from mental disorder of any description and other persons aged eighteen or over who are substantially and permanently handicapped by illness, injury or congenital deformity or such other disabilities as may be prescribed by the minister'.

7

Living in communal settings

Collective living arrangements are unusual and particularly so in Britain where, this chapter will suggest, there is some hostility to 'communitaire' philosophies. Living together with others of roughly the same age or generation is a feature of life for some people in student halls of residence or in other forms of shared housing at the beginning of adulthood but does not become so again until some 50 or 60 years later in specialized housing provision or in residential or nursing care. At either end of the adult life course it is very much a minority experience. However, the two living arrangements are perceived very differently. At the young end, communal living is seen as exciting and vibrant, albeit with its downside, but as far as later life is concerned it is generally viewed negatively. In between the two extremes communal living is even more a minority experience intended either for people under pensionable age with 'special needs' or for small groups of people who espouse 'alternative' lifestyles and opt to live collectively.

How do we define communal living for older people? We mean living arrangements where there is some degree or other of communal or public space and some degree or other of sharing of facilities. Within this definition, therefore, we include specialist housing provision, which in Britain is often known as sheltered housing, and care provision, namely residential or nursing care. (For the purposes of this discussion living in hospital provision is excluded. Also the term residential care will include nursing care unless specified otherwise.) The boundary between the two forms of communal living has been quite distinct until fairly recently. Where housing provision is concerned, residents have their 'own front door'. They are householders with housing rights and care and support is, largely, an add-on. With care provision the degree of communal living and sharing is greater and the residents are not independent householders. Care is an integral element. The chapter focuses largely on those communal arrangements for older people which have the characteristics of housing provision. However, as a key argument of the chapter is that the boundary between sheltered housing and residential care is becoming blurred and that definitions of what is housing and what is care are problematic, there will be some attention paid to residential care.

The numbers of older people living in communal living arrangements is small. Around 5 per cent of people aged 65 or over in Britain lived in sheltered housing in 1994 and a further 5 per cent lived in housing with a non-resident warden (Tinker *et al.* 1999). Around 5 per cent of all older people aged over 65, but 20 per cent of those over 85, live in residential care homes, nursing homes or hospital. Despite these low numbers the interest in communal living has been considerable. As we noted in Chapter 4, residential care has largely been seen as the provision of last resort in the context of a consistent policy focus, common to all political parties, to maintain people in their own homes wherever possible (Means and Smith 1998a). As far as specialized housing provision is concerned there has been a particularly lively debate between researchers about sheltered housing; a debate which at times in the past has become almost heated and during which at least one participant, Oldman, has arguably changed sides! The essential feature about these different debates about collective living arrangements for older people is that the latter have not, in any fundamental sense, been active participants.

The chapter aims to do two things. It documents past, present and likely future developments in housing and care provision and also reviews critically the arguments and assumptions that have accompanied these developments. The chapter starts by outlining a framework for evaluating the range of different communal living arrangements. The discussion here very much links back to the arguments presented in Chapter 2 about independent living and the meaning of home. The chapter then looks at residential care and in more detail at specialized housing provision. It moves on to draw on research by Oldman and others on recent and innovative developments in housing and care provision. The penultimate section of the chapter looks at what is known about older people's perceptions on communal living and particularly on their views of the newer forms of housing with care provision. The chapter concludes that policy development has largely neglected the social and collective dimension of later life.

Definitions and debates

Significantly, in the English language there is no equivalent concept for the French phrase *hebergement collectif*. In the UK policy and research literature, collective living is equated with institutional care and is contrasted unfavourably with living at home. Residential homes have been portrayed as exemplifying institutional life. Institutional care is where individuals spend the bulk of their sleeping and waking time in a setting which is not *their* home (Higgins 1989). Higgins has proposed an institution/at home dichotomy reproduced in Table 7.1. It is a valuable 'ideal type', against which the different living arrangements discussed in the chapter can be evaluated. In this model the characteristics of home and institution are polar, for example public/private space and strangeness of people/familiarity of people.

Table 7.1 Key characteristics of institutions and home

Institutions	*Home*
1 Public space, limitations in privacy	1 Private space but may be some limitations in privacy
2 Living with strangers, rarely alone	2 May live alone or with relatives or friends, rarely with strangers
3 Staffed by professionals or volunteers	3 Normally no staff but they may visit to provide services
4 Formal and lacking in intimacy	4 Informal and intimate
5 Sexual relationships discouraged	5 Sexual relationships (between certain family members) accepted
6 Owned or rented by other agencies	6 Owned and rented by inhabitants
7 Variations in size but may be large (in terms of physical space and numbers living in them)	7 Variations in size but usually small
8 Limitations on choice and on personal freedom	8 Ability to exercise choice and considerable degree of freedom
9 Strangeness (of people, place, etc.)	9 Familiarity (of people, place, etc.)
10 Batch or communal living	10 Individual arrangements for eating, sleeping, leisure activities which can vary according to time and place

Source: Higgins 1989: 15

Higgins is in a long line of researchers (T. Booth 1985; Hughes and Wilkin 1987; Willcocks *et al.* 1987) who have been influenced by theoretical critiques of institutions such as those of Goffman (1961) and Foucault (1967, 1977). Higgins' batch living is taken from Goffman's famous analysis of life in total institutions. Very largely, researchers have been uninterested in residential care as a form of housing/accommodation; it is not perceived as an example of communal or shared housing. The inherent assumption (we noted in Chapter 2) is that living at home is infinitely a more positive experience than living in a home. It offers privacy, informality, freedom and familiarity. Peace and colleagues (1997) in their reappraisal of residential care conducted some ten years after their study of local authority residential care (Willcocks *et al.* 1987) acknowledged that some residential care has tried to take on the characteristic of domestic environments in response to concerns about low standards and the depersonalizing effects of institutional living. They concluded, however, that 'Older people are still wary. We have argued that this wariness is justified in so far as residential settings still represent a threat not to individuality but, much more profoundly, to the sense of self' (Peace *et al.* 1997: 122).

Traditionally, sheltered housing has been portrayed as 'independent living' while residential care represents dependent living. Higgins (1989) herself did not position sheltered housing in the right-hand side of her table; for her it possessed some of the characteristics of an institution. However, quite clearly, the various forms of housing with care which will be reviewed in this chapter do not easily fit neatly into the left-hand side either. A central aim of the discussion is to explore the extent to which these forms are quasi-institution or quasi-home.

Residential care: issues and trends

History

The present system of residential care evolves directly from the Poor Law traditions of the nineteenth and early twentieth centuries. The opportunity espoused by Beveridge and Bevan immediately after the war to provide a comfortable, attractive, 'hotel model' of provision was never implemented. The local authority home was set up by the National Assistance Act 1948. Section 21 stated that it shall be the duty of every local authority to provide residential accommodation for persons who 'by reasons of age, infirmity or any other circumstances are in need of care or attention which is not otherwise available'.

Chapter 4 showed that although since the 1950s policy rhetoric stressed the desirability of supporting older people in their own homes, there was very little progress made towards developing community care alternatives to residential care. As discussed in Chapter 4, the latter received an unintentional massive fillip in the 1980s when changes to the social assistance scheme allowed older people to enter private and voluntary sector (not local authority) residential care without any assessment of their need but solely on the basis of financial situation. A dramatic increase in residents of independent sector homes resulted.

The principal purpose of the NHS and Community Care Act 1990 was to remove the 'perverse incentive' in favour of residential care. It has been only partly successful. As soon as weekly home care costs more to social services than a week's residential care, a move into care becomes likely. Charging frameworks take into account the capital released from the sale of an older person's property when they enter residential care and a residential allowance is available from the government to fund individuals in private and voluntary nursing and residential homes. Increasing numbers of older people are home-owners (in part because of Conservative governments' right to buy policies). As a result, in nearly all situations it is substantially cheaper for local authorities to place people in residential care, even where there is no difference between the gross cost of residential care and care at home (Audit Commission 1996). Between 1970 and 1998, the overall number of residential care, nursing home and NHS long-stay places in the UK has more than doubled but the balance of provision has shifted dramatically in that period with local authority and NHS long-stay provision falling sharply, private residential care growing constantly and nursing homes the fastest growing sector.

Demand or need

Demand and need are problematic concepts as far as residential care is concerned. There is no agreed dependency level at which entry to a care home is assumed appropriate. There are a range of factors explaining why one person goes into a home and another does not. It is, for example, often commented that having a spouse is one of the most important factors keeping people out of care homes (Laing and Buisson 1998: 84). Care needs are a factor, but only one. Inappropriate housing may be a factor contributing to admission (Tinker *et al.* 1999). Netten *et al.* (1998) found that nearly half of all residential care residents had low dependency, 16 per cent had moderate dependency, 18 per cent had severe dependency and 20 per cent had total dependency.[1]

The idea of demand in relation to residential care is not much discussed. Much of the debate in Britain concerning long-term care for older people has been about its funding system and the faultlines that flow from that system. There has been insufficient attention paid to a significant minority of current residents who are outside the system.[2] An estimated 29 per cent of all residents in residential care and 27 per cent in nursing homes are private payers, responsible for all of the costs (Royal Commission 1999). Oldman and Quilgars (1999) focused on self-payers in a study of residential care and showed that for some the notion of 'demand' was real enough. For some the move, contrary to conventional wisdom, had been a positive choice and it had been a decision they had been in control of. They reported that they were less lonely and less bored than they had been prior to the move, trapped as they had been in their homes. Oldman and Quilgars' study also suggested that admission to a home does not necessarily signal a loss of independence for either self-payers or local authority funded residents but that the latter were less able to exercise any choice in the decision. *Demand* is not a solid concept for those needing public subsidies. Rather, the focus is on care *needs* and how they can be most cost effectively met. The idea that collective living may be sought is not typically part of public sector assessments. The concept of choice is illusory for those without substantial financial resources. While a majority would prefer to remain at home but are unable to do so, a minority who do 'demand' residential care, are denied the opportunity to move to communal arrangements.

It is possible for people's quality of life to improve as a consequence of a move to residential care. The prevailing negative attitude to communal living in general and residential care in particular is not entirely helpful. Moving into a home is seen as loss of independence even as some sort of failure. A Department of Health (1994a) report titled *The F Factor: Reasons Why Some Older People Choose Residential Care* asked the question why it was that some people managed to remain in the community but others *failed*. The very measures which would make residential homes more acceptable, such as the exercise of more control over the decision by a prospective resident, or the use of residential homes by a larger section of the population, are ruled out. Two potentially conflicting processes exist alongside each other, the one to promote residential care as a positive resource to be used only as the option of a choice, the other to keep people out of residential homes for as long as possible (Clough 1997).

Most older people, prior to a move, are no different from the rest of society in their attitude to residential care. Oldman and Quilgars' study included a

group of older people, living in mainstream housing, who had been designated as on 'the margins of residential care'. The following comment from
one of this group is typical of a prevailing attitude:

> I just didn't want to go into care . . . if I go into a home I've got a horror of
> sitting around waiting, doing nothing and you lose all your independence
> whereas here [a sheltered flat] I've got my own home and I can do my
> own things . . . shut my own front door. I've still got my own life,
> that's what I was afraid of losing. I would like to think I was going to
> stay here as long as I can.
>
> (Oldman and Quilgars 1999: 372)

Some of those who had moved into a home, however, expressed very different views; life had become more interesting, less stressful and more sociable.
Some gained, not lost independence. A relative, who said she had been
surprised that her mother had been so positive, commented: 'I think she
was glad to move into a home because she had to rely on us and she has
always hated having to do that' (Oldman and Quilgars 1999: 376).

However, residential care is increasingly targeted at the very frail: an estimated 20 per cent of residents have some form of dementia (Royal Commission 1999). Such trends impact adversely on those older people who are trying
to seek out the benefits of communal living. In the Oldman and Quilgars
study, not everyone felt their expectations of an improved quality of life
had been met: 'Most of the old people here are senile old women. I can't
talk to them like I do to you' (Oldman and Quilgars 1999: 380).

Current issues

At the time of writing this chapter, the system of regulation of social care in
the UK is being radically changed via the Care Standards Act 2000 (to be
implemented in 2002). At present private and voluntary residential and
nursing homes must be registered under the Residential Homes Act (RHA)
1984. If a living arrangement is providing personal care and meals it is obliged
to register under the RHA and then fall under the responsibilities of the social
care regulatory authorities. Under the new arrangements registration, inspection and enforcement will be extended to local authorities' own care homes
and statutory regulation of domiciliary care introduced for the first time.
The new National Care Standards Commission will be established to take over
the regulation of care services from individual local and health authorities.

The Royal Commission on Long Term Care (Royal Commission 1999) was
enormously influential in drawing attention to the current issues bedevilling
care provision. Those who move into residential or nursing care commonly do
so in their mid-eighties, often after the trauma of an admission to hospital or a
period of living at home with care services. There is great deal of concern and
anxiety about the funding arrangements, which are perceived to be unfair.
Many older people believe they are made to pay twice, once through the
national insurance system which they thought would pay for their needs
in later life and again out of their assets. Older people who own their own

property have to use their assets to pay for their care. Those who are funded by the state are left with only a small sum as 'pocket money'. The inequity between free NHS care and social care for which charges are levied is a growing concern with the withdrawal of long-term care from the NHS. If an older person has cancer they will receive care free at the point of consumption; if they suffer from Alzheimer's they might be paying in excess of £350 a week in a nursing home. The current funding system provides no incentive to local authorities to provide domiciliary care. The system appears to be designed around a series of different bureaucracies rather than the needs of individual older people.

Lastly, to end on a more positive note, physical standards in homes have improved, for example an increase in single rooms and rooms with an en suite toilet. Quality assurance is in vogue and standards in the quality of care have become more transparent. In a small number of developments, living arrangements have become more home like (where residents live in flatlets with their own bathroom, small kitchen and their own front door with a bell and letter box). In the future there might be possibilities for far more radical changes. The Royal Commission noted in passing that residents in some developments in Denmark are not stripped of their assets but lease units which can be sold after death. Such initiatives could be imported to the UK.

Sheltered housing: issues and trends

The development of sheltered housing

> sheltered housing's origins lie in a social housing response to older people's needs that predate community care policy by almost 40 years.
> (Nocon and Pleace 1999: 167)

It will be quite apparent at this point in the book that there is no single policy for care and accommodation for older people, notwithstanding the community care reforms in the early 1990s. The two types of communal living come from different routes. It is only now at the beginning of the twenty-first century that there is some evidence of convergence.

Sheltered housing in its current form goes back as far as the 1950s (Butler *et al.* 1983) and shortly after, sometime in the 1960s, the debate began about whether it was meeting housing need or care need. At this point sheltered housing was quite clearly seen as an alternative to the sort of demeaning and sometimes abusive residential care which Townsend (1962) was so effectively inveighing against in his now famous study *The Last Refuge*. At the same time local authority housing departments saw the development of sheltered housing as an opportunity to address their general housing responsibilities. At a time of housing need, older people were seen as under-occupying council houses which were sorely needed for families. If older people could be attracted by the offer of small, purpose-built manageable accommodation with some support, a larger housing problem could be solved. In the 1970s as public expenditure crises loomed, sheltered housing gained even more in popularity as it became increasingly apparent that residential care was expensive and being used for significant numbers of older people who did not need it (Plank 1977; Neill *et al.* 1988). As Chapter 2 noted, the concept of the continuum of care held sway at this time and policy analysts were enjoined with the task of devising resource allocation models which would ensure that people moved to a more intensive stage when a specified level of dependency had been reached.

The current official unpopularity of sheltered housing was kicked off by academics in the 1980s; policy commentators caught up rather later. Butler *et al.* (1983) also questioned some of the claims made by providers of sheltered housing and particularly sneered over what they labelled the dog food model, that is the claim that it 'prolonged' life. Laura Middleton (1981) in her research equally criticized the provision, employing the epithet *So much for so few*. Middleton was critical of the segregation from the rest of the community, which she believed the provision embodied. It was a myth, she claimed, that it helped maintain independent living when it involved moving to a community under surveillance. In a similar vein, Clapham and various colleagues have condemned sheltered housing on the grounds that it is 'special needs' and stigmatizing. Clapham and Munro (1988) argued for sheltered housing resources to be made available to the wider community in which it is located. Clapham has argued that sheltered housing was ill thought out and over provided and should be brought fully into the mainstream of community care through upgrading to very sheltered standards (Clapham and Munro 1990; Clapham 1997).

During the 1980s and 1990s sheltered housing providers began to address the various management problems that they were then facing. Tenant populations were ageing and morbidity levels increasing. The limited facilities of sheltered housing provided insufficient support and domiciliary care was often unavailable or inadequate. Wardens complained that they were subject to severe work pressures. At this time the provision was generally not claiming to provide a 'home for life'. There was evidence that moves to residential care from sheltered housing were greater than for equivalent populations living in mainstream housing (McCafferty 1994; Royal Commission 1999). Providers were able to access on behalf of their tenants the entitlement-based means-tested residential care allowance. In addition, on-site wardens were able to exert some pressure locally to achieve a move for tenants who were making their jobs burdensome. After the changes to the funding of residential care in April 1993, it became harder to move tenants to residential care because social services had to be persuaded of the need. All these various developments were the driver behind the emergence at this time of very sheltered housing. The latter is distinguishable from 'ordinary' sheltered housing as follows:

- the provision of a meal
- the provision of additional services
- the possibility of a more barrier-free environment.

A further issue was that of 'difficult to let' sheltered housing. In 1994 8 per cent of local authority and 13 per cent of housing associations had over half their stock designated as difficult to let. Tinker *et al.*'s (1995) explanations for this phenomenon were undesirable locations, too small accommodation including unpopular bed-sits, sharing of some facilities and lack of facilities such as lifts. Tinker *et al.* (1995) also found that very sheltered housing was not exempt from the 'difficult to let' problem. Other commentators (Oldman 1991b; Marsh and Riseborough 1995; Nocon and Pleace 1999) have suggested that affordability, the perception that high rents and service charges are not giving value for money, is a further reason for the difficulty some providers have had in filling schemes.

By the 1990s sheltered housing was falling out of favour at the policy centre in part because of the government's commitment to 'new' community care principles and in part because of pressures to reduce public expenditure. As Chapters 4 and 5 have shown, the strong message from several quarters starting with the White Paper *Caring for People* (DoH 1989) was that older people should be supported in their own, existing, homes where, it was stated, they preferred to be. Initiatives such as Care and Repair were heavily promoted at the expense of moving options, although it must be noted that the promotion was mostly of the rhetorical variety. The Care and Repair movement has always received scant financial rewards from governments.

Special needs housing, or to use its more acceptable label supported housing, lost a lot of popularity as the new era, heralded by the NHS and Community Care Act 1990, swept in. Cooper *et al.* (1994) commented:

> The image of shared housing has . . . suffered from the declining importance attached to the idea of communality and the growing emphasis on independent living and personal autonomy as the central goal of supported housing.
>
> (Cooper *et al.* 1994: 3)

The *Living Independently* study (McCafferty 1994) was critical of the fact that sheltered housing was accommodating high levels of low dependency. A key finding was that a high proportion of recent entrants (41 per cent of ordinary sheltered housing tenants and 22 per cent of very sheltered housing tenants) had no physical or mental dependency. Finally the Audit Commission (1998) waded in with its quite influential report *Home Alone*.

> The principle of community care makes it harder to justify tying resources to property rather than people. Sheltered housing must accordingly re-invent itself as provision for older people who prefer the presence of a supportive community or it must re-think the levels of need it is able to support. If it does not it will face serious questions about its relevance in a system which can deliver high levels of support in ordinary housing.
>
> (Audit Commission 1998: 28)

Essentially, the new community care is driven by concerns about public expenditure. The major explanation for sheltered housing's current lack of popularity is its perceived cost. We have already noted the dramatic decline in capital subsidies available for specialized housing provision for older people. The supply of sheltered housing as measured by new completions fell dramatically, Chapter 5 notes, in the local authority, housing association and private sectors alike.

The warden and Supporting People

This discussion of the history of sheltered housing finishes with two related topics, the 'warden' and *Supporting People* (DSS 1998b). The warden is, arguably, the sine qua non of sheltered housing and her role has been endlessly argued over. Wardens' contractual obligations have always excluded the delivery of care yet in their 'good neighbour' role of yesteryear they have been inevitably drawn into activities that get categorized as 'hands-on care'. The new role that is being asked of sheltered housing has involved a shift in the role of the warden from good neighbour to one that emphasizes enabling and coordinating. Providers and wardens alike have welcomed the new professionalism that this implies (Hasler and Page 1998; Thompson and Page 1999). However, there is evidence (England *et al.* 2000) that the role of the warden continues to be confused. Relatives and warden are not clear what wardens do and the respective responsibilities of warden and relatives are muddled. In the context of the new community care, wardens are moving away from their direct contact, good neighbour role to one of manager, co-ordinator and professional. For tenants and relatives there is a paradox. At a time when sheltered housing is claiming to support people with care needs, wardens are perceived to have less direct contact with tenants.

The role of the warden is exemplary of the long-standing policy confusion over what is a housing/care/support activity. In 2003 the government will introduce the new policy and funding regime for sheltered and supported housing (*Supporting People*) to resolve, among other things, these difficulties. Housing benefit service charges will no longer be available to fund the care and support element of supported housing. Instead, there will be introduced a new cash-limited, needs-assessed grant administered by local commissioning panels. Currently the warden service is a very significant element of the expenditure on housing benefit service charges (Cebulla *et al.* 1999). It is not at all clear whether the new commissioning panels will be prepared to fund the sort of preventive, low-level support service carried out by sheltered housing wardens to the same level as now. Also it is not clear whether *Supporting People* represents a threat or an opportunity to housing and care provision, dependent as it currently is on housing benefit as a major source of financial support.

Sheltered housing's development has been characterized by a general absence of older people themselves from debates about its different variants. Before we put the older person centre stage, we look more closely at the apparent blurring of boundaries between housing and care.

Blurring the boundaries between housing and care: very sheltered housing

The once sharp divide between 'housing' and 'care' has recently been breached. There are now emerging, albeit in very limited numbers,[3] models of provision which conform neither to pure sheltered housing nor pure residential care. The blurring is coming from two directions. Residential care is becoming more 'homely' and sheltered housing more institutional.

Although, as Tinker *et al.* (1999) have commented, very sheltered housing has been around since the late 1970s, since the mid-1990s or so there has been a surge of interest in hybrid forms of provision variously called very sheltered housing, assisted living, close care, category two and a half.[4] The new century has seen a spate of conferences and publications about housing forms of provision for older people which, the protagonists claim, promote independence and dignity and reduce reliance on residential care. In some areas of Britain, the impetus for new forms of very sheltered housing have come from social services departments faced with problems caused by old and outmoded local authority homes. There have also been other developments which have contributed to the recent interest in the potential of housing based schemes to support frail older people. The Royal Commission on Long Term Care called for further expansion and development of innovative housing schemes. Very sheltered housing was one of four alternatives to residential care which the Commission singled out for specialized study and comparative costing.[5] In addition, the Department of Health with the White Paper *Modernising Social Services* (DoH 1998a) and subsequent guidance put considerable emphasis on prevention, independence and, by implication, on alternatives to residential care. Increasingly strong claims are being made that residential care is outdated and unlikely to survive in the long term and can be replaced by housing models. There is also a view that housing-based schemes are a better solution than traditional residential care for dementia sufferers, although most providers are uneasy about accommodating the confused with the not confused (for example, the eveidence given by the Association of Directors of Social Services to the Royal Commission).

The analysis of the blurring of boundaries between housing and care which follows is based on research by Oldman (2000b). There are a number of key issues. These are whether a scheme is registered or not, whether the accommodation and care are provided by the same organization or not, whether the scheme provides independent living and whether a home for life is guaranteed and finally whether very sheltered housing is a cost-effective alternative to residential care.

Registration

The sales appeal of housing-based models is that occupants have their 'own front door'. Many proponents set great store by the fact that older people have their own tenancies or leases. They have security of tenure and their rights are enshrined in housing law. Schemes are intended to feel more like living 'at home' than 'living in a home' (Oldman and Quilgars 1999). A central issue is whether the 'housing' nature of a model is compromised if the scheme is registered under the Residential Homes Act 1984, which it may be required to do because it offers board and care. In a registered scheme the older person has the status of licensee not tenant and as such they are not entitled to housing benefit and other community benefits.

The Residential Homes Act has been subject to local differences in interpretation. An identical very sheltered housing scheme may be required to have been registered in one part of Britain but not in another. Many very sheltered housing providers aim to 'avoid' registration although ironically before the April 1993 changes in the funding of residential care housing schemes would purposefully seek registration in order to access the residential care allowance (Clapham *et al.* 1994). The main reasons for wanting to avoid registration are the increased bureaucracy and increased costs that housing providers believe come in its wake. It is also argued that principles of independent living are threatened by the requirements of registration which make, it is argued, a scheme more institutional in feel.

There has been little discussion in the field of housing provision for older people about what Steve Griffiths (1997) has called the pauperization effect of registration on occupants. An older person living in residential care, entitled to financial support from the state with fees, is left with the personal allowance of £15.45 (April 2000 to April 2001) a week. If the scheme was deregistered the same person would be entitled to attendance allowance/disability living allowance and income support/housing benefit additions for severe disability and older age. Disposable income could increase to up to £100 a week, out of which, however, the older person would then have to pay for food, light, heating, laundry and care.

In Oldman's research some providers argued that registration would seriously damage their service delivery philosophy. Quality of care, they argued, could be monitored in other ways, principally through contract compliance. Other providers had different views; some believed that service provision for frail older people had to be approached differently from provision for other groups. Issues of protection were central, it was believed. One provider said 'We need the safeguard of regulation'. Another provider felt strongly that the issue of registration could be something of a red herring. Principles of empowerment and independent living were independent of legal definitions. Registered schemes were capable of being liberating environments. Equally non-registered schemes could be disempowering and institutional in feel.

Integration/separation of accommodation and care support

Within the supported housing movement there is generally a view that vulnerable people have a better chance to live empowered lives if their landlord and their care/support deliverers are different organizations. Schemes, it is argued, are more likely to feel like ordinary housing and less like residential care. Simons (1998) has noted that the key defining feature of residential care is not the provision of personal care but the way in which the place in which people live is inextricably bound up with the help they receive.

Simons' expertise lies largely in the field of learning disability. He argues that separating care from accommodation gives more control and power to residents or tenants. The latter can sack their care provider without fear of losing their accommodation. As far as provision for older people is concerned, the debate about whether accommodation or care should be separate is rarely conducted in these terms but much more in terms of the perceived cost-effectiveness of the two different arrangements or linked to the arguments about registration. If accommodation and care are provided by the same organization, registration may be required.

Home for life/ageing in situ

All of the models reviewed had some degree of commitment to the principle of continuing care; this is what distinguished them from ordinary sheltered housing. However, the extent to which this is a central aim or is made explicit and transparent differs from model to model. In some the claim is to provide care up to and including nursing care.

It was apparent from the study that the issue of home for life is problematic and needs considerable clarification. Explicit policies on home for life seemed largely absent. In most non-registered schemes residents are assured tenants and hence have security of tenure. However, movement to residential and nursing care was evident in many of the schemes under investigation. It was not always clear in what circumstances this was happening and who was the key decision maker: landlord, GP or other health professional, older person or family member. Respondents' usual response was to say: 'There is no general rule about this. We have to look at each individual circumstance'.

Dementia presented the chief difficulty to managers. Where the lives of other residents were perceived to be adversely affected by the behaviour or actions of someone with a dementia condition, a move to nursing or residential care was often strongly encouraged.

Independent living

It is said that very sheltered housing is different from and better than residential care because it is not based on a dependency model. Respondents who claimed that they were providing an alternative to residential care would commonly assert that their service delivery was underpinned by a philosophy that stressed independence and marked out what they were doing from what might be found in a standard residential home:

> There is every sign that extraCare is capable of evolving into a realistic alternative to the care provided in residential or nursing homes for the great majority of older people needing some form of grouped provision. It has the great advantage of not carrying the stigma of an institution, of making possible a greater degree of independence and self determination and offering older people much more generous private space and offering older people much more generous private space as a basis for

the fulfilment of all the other rights individuals should be able to enjoy.
(Greenwood and Smith 1999: 37)

The challenge for an evaluator is to test out these claims. Does the concept of
'own front door', housing rights and the ethos of 'independent living' result in
an environment which feels like living 'at home' not 'in a home'. Has 'institutional drift' highlighted as a potential problem by Age Concern been avoided
(Age Concern 1998)?

Almost all respondents, regardless of the explicit aims of the scheme, said
that they tried to promote independence and encourage residents to do things
for themselves. Some stressed the flexibility of their service; for example the
amount of care received might be increased after an illness or after a period
in hospital but reduced again when more independence was regained. Most
schemes employed the now well-established practices of care management:
care plans, reviews and key workers.

Cheaper than residential care?

A number of contentious claims have been made about the cost-effectiveness
of very sheltered housing. When very sheltered housing is claimed to be
cheaper than other forms of care the question must be asked: *cheaper to
whom?* Social services departments, for example, have benefited by the
adoption of very sheltered housing since costs can then be shunted to other
budgets, namely the housing benefit budget and in some cases to tenants'
personal budgets. Most costing exercises do not include the help provided
by informal carers.

The Royal Commission on Long Term Care, using costings employed by
Ernst and Young (1994) and Netten and Dennett (1997), concluded that
there is no general rule about whether care in ordinary housing costs more
or less than care in very sheltered housing or full-time residential care.
It depends instead on how many hours home care, including day and night
sitting are needed and how far such care is provided by the staff of very
sheltered housing.

The user perspective on communal living arrangements

How do older people view communal living arrangements? The following
discussion is based on demand information, empirical research and the experiences of other countries.

Demand data

Where is the evidence that some older people do not have the same negative
attitude to living with each other that the 'not old' world generally has?
Waiting lists to local authority and housing association housing schemes are
testimony to some sort of a demand for such living. Even Tinker (1989;
Tinker *et al.* 1995, 1999) and McCafferty (1994), as unhappy as they are
about the emphasis in the past given to housing need not care needs, confirm

the popularity of the provision. This book is not in any way denying findings concerning schemes that are difficult to let or concerning the significant minority of tenants who would have preferred to have stayed in their own homes. But there is evidence that although older people share the rest of the world's antipathy to the workhouse image of residential care, *some* choose to move to what academics call 'age segregated' communities. The evidence is there from enquiry lines to all the main national and local older people's advice lines, from the quite considerable numbers of older owner-occupiers who despite the house price crisis at the end of the 1980s continued to purchase retirement housing, from social housing landlord registers and, finally (we see below) from *some* research studies.

Empirical research on the new perspective

Nocon and Pleace (1999) carried out for Shropshire housing officers a large user study involving focus groups as well as individual interviews. They found that people had moved because they wanted company, more security, freedom from worry about housing, and a better quality of life than they had before. They wanted to escape neighbourhoods which, once supportive, were no longer congenial. They highly valued the practical support they got from wardens. They did not really want to talk about care needs and care plans. What was more salient for the older people in the study was everyday life, having enough to do and going out. The researchers concluded:

> The isolation and the difficulty of organising things for yourself that can accompany age or vulnerability are often among the worst elements of the experience of ill health or frailty, even if basic care needs met. Sheltered housing, judging by the results of the research can help to overcome some of the fears and concerns experienced by older people and can thereby help to improve their quality of life.
>
> (Nocon and Pleace 1999: 178)

The focus of England *et al.*'s (2000) study was the role of relatives in sheltered housing. Equal prominence was given to the views of tenants, wardens and relatives. Tenants stressed the mutual support they gave each other and freedom they felt from being less dependent on relatives. All three parties talked about the notion of sheltered housing as village, they all stressed the social interactions which constitute social housing living and the importance of social relationships as a form of social support.

What older people think of very sheltered housing

Oldman (2000b) attempted to obtain a user perspective on the new forms of provision where boundaries between housing and care are blurring. Interviews were organized around four themes:

- What sort of place is this, institution or home; what does the concept of 'your own front door' mean to you?

- Independent living, what does that mean?
- Affordability.
- Relationships with relatives.

The objective was to operationalize Higgins' (1989) typology presented at the beginning of this chapter by finding out whether very sheltered schemes people were living in felt like 'living at home' or 'living in a home'. Higgins' ten ideal type factors which describe institution and home are immensely useful in appraising living arrangements which are quasi-home or quasi-institution. Here we discuss just two of these: 'number one: space and privacy' and 'number eight: choice'. The relationship between public space and privacy is complex. Where there is a great deal of emphasis on privacy sociability can be a casualty. The schemes which were most liked were those where people felt at ease with the balance of private and public space. Choice too is problematic. The most highly valued places were where tenants had been completely free to choose what help they wanted (Clarke *et al.* 1998).

The degree to which a scheme did feel like home seemed to be a function of the choice that people felt they had had in moving in. Access to most schemes was tightly controlled. Allocation policies were based on the premise that the new hybrid forms of provision are scarce resources and should be targeted at those most in need; in many cases panels made up of representatives of social services, housing department and provider were employed. But schemes most felt like home where people felt their desire for group living had been met; however, in many cases assessment criteria ignored social and collective needs. Schemes also felt more like home when providers tried to achieve what has been called 'balanced communities'. There were lower levels of satisfaction when providers allocated all their tenancies to 'high dependency' applicants. Furthermore there was a dissonance between older people and providers about when to move to schemes. The latter wanted to focus on the most needy; most of the older people in the study felt that it was better to move before the onset of weariness and extreme disability.

Schemes had objectives which were in conflict; on the one hand they purported to enhance quality of life, to rehabilitate and to prevent but on the other they also claimed to replace or divert from residential care. Those schemes which put more emphasis on the former than the latter were enjoyed more than those that were reinventions of residential care different only in boasting 'your own front door'. Phrases on the lines of 'I am a different person now', 'My friends don't recognize me', 'I am less depressed and unhappy' were quite common. Despite poor health, reduced income and the loss of partners and friends from an earlier time, if people could find a kindred spirit and they had enough to do and the staff just helped them rather than administered care plans, they could be well satisfied with their living arrangements. In those schemes with a mix of dependencies mutual support was in evidence. Living in a place where everybody was highly disabled at point of moving in was not liked.

Simply giving people their 'own front door' did not achieve independent living, although schemes which were registered and hence people did not have tenancy rights seemed less liked than non-registered schemes. As

Chapter 2 suggested, independent living is a complex phrase and means different things to different people. Where high levels of care are being delivered to schemes, the danger is that the place becomes an institution. Twigg's (1997) contention that carers behave less obtrusively and in a less ageist manner when delivering care to people's homes as opposed to 'a home' was only partly borne out in the study. Ageist attitudes by care givers were in evidence and institutional drift a danger.

The affordability of very sheltered living has been the least researched aspect of the provision. Affordability is a complex issue and was contingent on many factors, income and wealth of the tenant, whether informal care constituted a significant part of someone's total support package, their level of disability and so on. Non-registered schemes give people higher disposable incomes and, it was quite evident, feelings of some power and control.

What marks out residential care from housing-based models is the involvement of relatives in the latter. Family members are called 'informal carers' when they provide care and support to older people living in ordinary housing in the community. When family members visit older people in residential care they are referred to as 'relatives' because it is assumed they have largely abdicated the task of caring to professional carers. The key defining characteristic of very sheltered housing seemed to revolve around relatives. Where older people had relatives, the latter were very involved and were a major factor in a disabled person's ability to keep going. Relatives said they felt that the older person's move to the very sheltered scheme had enabled them to keep going as a carer, 'to go the last mile'.

Other countries' models

In mainland Europe, with its very different welfare and housing traditions from the UK, there is a more positive approach to collective living arrangements. In addition, attitudes are a little different, a little less paternalistic and in some European countries older people are a significant and sometimes potent political force. Brenton (1998) has looked at the possibilities of importing the Dutch co-housing model to the UK. There are 200 such groups in the Netherlands where a wide range of age groups have opted to live together as part of a group where each have their own private dwelling. They remain in charge of their lives, are free to make choices to live with whom they choose and in a way they choose. One resident is quoted: 'It is important to move while you still can to a place you choose before other people move you to a place they choose' (Brenton 1998: 1).

At the present moment in the UK there is nothing resembling co-housing for older people although Joseph Rowntree Foundation's continuing community Hartrigg Oaks in New Earswick, near York, is an example of where like-minded people have opted to live together (Rugg 1999).

Conclusion

The chapter has charted the development of communal living arrangements in Britain for older people. It has shown that they have evolved along quite separate lines – residential care on the one hand and sheltered housing in its various forms on the other. Now there is some evidence of a blurring of the boundaries between the two. Residential care in very modest ways is becoming more domestic and less institutional; sheltered housing is moving much further along the care continuum. Indeed some commentators have gone so far as to predict the end of traditional residential care and a move to a model where everyone has their 'own front door'.

In Britain we tend to look very negatively at collective living arrangements in later life, seeing them as unavoidable for those for whom it is no longer cost-effective to support in their own homes. Older people are allowed to move to schemes only when their very frailty makes it difficult for them to derive much benefit from collective arrangements. In this book we have generally welcomed the recent closer integration of housing with community care, but it brings its dangers. The emergence of hybrid forms of provision – the 'blurring of boundaries' – has to be welcomed in some ways. At last we are moving away from the old workhouse image of residential care which has persisted so long. But the closer integration of housing and care (as Chapter 2 noted) does not represent a conversion by providers and policy makers to genuine notions of independent living, to concepts of empowerment and self-determination. The phrase 'independent living' really is a smokescreen. Behind it lives on the medical model, activities of daily living, care planning and assessment. The blurring of boundaries between housing and care can illustrate the downside of joint working discussed in Chapter 8. Joint working allows resources to be combined and Best Value to be delivered. Best Value, however, in the area of policies for older people, can miss what older people themselves value.

The chapter has suggested that older people are social animals like everybody else. Some have become depressed at living in now alienating environments, with very little to do and very few people to talk to. It is to miss the point to suggest that the benefits of sheltered housing and low-level practical support can be grafted on to older people's existing homes. They can, but the concept of a viable community where some quality of life can be regained cannot.

What grounds are there for optimism that we can move away from the dominant medical model of disability which underpins housing and care provision to one that more resembles the vision sketched out by Brenton (1998) in her discussion of the transferability of the Dutch co-housing model to the UK? The climate seems propitious; the rhetoric is one of empowerment and citizenship (Fletcher *et al.* 1999). Older people are being listened to; they are being involved. The 'baby boomers' (Evandrou 1997) will have opportunities and attitudes that are quite different from today's 80 and 90 year olds. The concept of direct payments have now been extended to older people. Rising and substantial levels of equity may mean that the Royal Commission's ideas about leasing residential care may become a reality.

In the short term, however, there are impending policy developments which threaten the above. First, the new regulation regime looks set to bring housing and care models into its embrace with consequent problems about low disposable incomes, pauperization and institutional drift. Second, the *Supporting People* regime, while it may oil the wheels of joint working between housing, health and social care, with its implicit hostility to collective living, may continue to threaten ideals of mutual support, empowerment and self-determination which are the hallmarks of positive communal living. Third, while residential care is improving, the continued driving down of the price of care and the consequent low profit margins means that providers have little scope to develop a wider range of amenities and more personalized care. Fourth, the unfairness which surrounds the funding of residential care continues.

Finally, this chapter has not been about the majority of older people. They want to live and die in the home they have probably lived in for some time. However, for a minority, living with other older people may not be anathema.

Notes

1 Barthel index of activities of daily living (grouped).
2 Under the means test, people with assets above £16,000 get no help with fees from either the social assistance scheme or the local authority. Assets of between £10,000 and £16,000 are assumed to generate a notional income of £1 per week per £250 of capital and this notional income is taken into account in the means test. Assets below £10,000 are disregarded. Income is also taken into account.
3 Laing and Buisson (1997) identified 17,000 such clients in the social rented sector.
4 In the discussion that follows we shall use the phrase 'very sheltered housing' in a generic sense to cover all the different housing and care models which have emerged in the last few years.
5 The other three were intensive home support, co-resident care and assistive technology.

8

Working together in the interests of older people?

The present Labour government places an enormous emphasis upon what it calls 'joined up thinking' between different agencies and different professionals. This is an emphasis clearly relevant to older people with their often complex needs, which cut across housing, health and social services. After some initial definitional work, this chapter outlines the present policy priority given by government to working together and where it does and does not relate to previous attempts to encourage collaborative working. The second half of the chapter draws on the involvement of two of us (Means and Heywood) in a large-scale exercise aimed to encourage effective joint working 'on the ground'. The result of this activity was the workbook *Making Partnerships Work in Community Care: A Guide for Practitioners in Housing, Health and Social Services* (Means *et al.* 1997), as official practice guidance by both the Department of Health and the DETR. The emphasis will be upon both the content of the book in terms of messages about joint working and the process of producing the book, which required a collaborative commitment from two government departments with no real history of joint working. Older people, of course, contribute by far the largest of community care priority groups. In any discussion on joint working, older people's needs will inevitably feature heavily. The effective delivery of an adaptations service (see Chapter 6), for example, requires good joint working between a number of different agencies. This chapter provides an analysis of all aspects of joint working.

What do we mean by working together?

It is very easy to assume that there is a consensus about what we mean by working together, and it is helpful to break down this definitional question by both level and activity. *Partnership in Action* (DoH 1998c) usefully distinguished the following three levels of joint working. At the strategic planning level, agencies need to plan jointly for the medium term, and share information about how they intend to use their resources towards the achievement of common goals. The second level was service commissioning which involved securing services for local populations and required agencies to have a common understanding of the needs they are jointly meeting, and the kind of provision likely to be most effective. Finally, in terms of service provision, service users want a coherent integrated package of care so that neither they nor their families face the anxiety of having to navigate a labyrinthine bureaucracy. This is regardless of how services are purchased or funded.

In terms of activity, it is possible to distinguish between a number of different levels of working together (Means *et al.* 1997), as follows.

Understanding each other

Joint working does not always involve meeting together. Professionals need to understand each other's agencies and so be able to advise their clients how these agencies might be able to help them. For example, mutual understanding is about a care manager having sufficient knowledge of housing to know when a joint assessment with housing is required because of the complexity of the housing and support issues to be tackled.

Cooperation

Professionals need a willingness to assist each other over individual cases in a constructive and positive manner, much of which cooperative interaction may well take place over the telephone. For example, this might involve a sheltered housing warden contacting health and social services on behalf of a resident with dementia.

Collaboration

Collaboration is when individual professionals or more often agencies begin to work together on specific issues, joint projects or shared cases. For example, this might involve housing, health and social services working together on a single regeneration budget bid to reduce the isolation of older people on an estate.

Coordination

Coordination involves a pan-agency attempt to work together to achieve agreed objectives. Although no formal partnership arrangement is signed, the coordination agreement may well be codified in written form. A joint protocol between housing and social services over referrals for very sheltered housing would be a good example of this.

Networks

Networks are informal gatherings of professionals who meet together to exchange views, improve mutual understanding and to develop cooperation and collaboration. They can often be a precursor to more formal coordination arrangements. Typical examples would be a neighbourhood forum for local field level staff from all the local agencies or a regular meeting of senior managers from health, housing and social services.

Partnership

Although it is sometimes used as a generic term (making partnerships work in housing, health and community care) partnership is increasingly reserved for formal, often contractual agreements along the lines required by the new Health Act 1999. The present Labour government expects health and social services to increasingly work in this way at both the strategic planning and service commissioning levels of joint working.

Involving older people in joint working

So far, the focus has been very much on professionals working together and yet the whole point of joint working at the strategic planning, service commissioning and service provision levels should be that it is a mechanism to ensure that appropriate housing, health and social services are made available to older people in need. One obvious way to ensure that this happens is to involve older people centrally in the joint working process, the importance of which has been stressed by central government in a number of initiatives such as tenant participation compacts (DETR 1999a) and Best Value (DETR 1998a). With regard to the latter, a key test of Best Value for local public services will be the views of service users and local taxpayers and the quality of consultation mechanisms designed to obtain those views.

The involvement of service users and older people in decision-making processes can take a number of forms. Drawing upon the work of d'Aboville (1994), it is possible to identify a spectrum of user involvement, outlined in Table 8.1, which spans from just providing information to full delegated

Table 8.1 Dimensions of user involvement

- Providing information to enable the older person to understand how to access services
- Individual consultation designed to enable service users to express their own needs and how they believe these could be best met
- Group consultation in which older people are consulted about what kinds of services are needed
- Service development input in which for example older service users may contribute to writing service specifications or setting quality assurance standards
- Delegated control in which statutory agencies hand over key decisions or actual services to individuals or to user-led organizations

---

control over services to user-led organizations. In looking at the spectrum in Table 8.1, it can be seen that it spans from minimal input to complete control of services, and that it covers involvement in joint working at both the strategic and operational levels. It also needs to be noted that delegated control can probably be set up only through joint working but that the end point is user control rather than inter-agency collaboration or partnership. The disability movement in the UK has demonstrated and frequently received involvement at the top end of the d'Aboville spectrum, and their goal has often been to minimize their dependence upon able-bodied professionals of any kind. Their critique of professionals will now be looked at and this will be followed by a consideration of its relevance to older people and joint working. This discussion on the disability *movement* should be linked with that in Chapter 2 on the social model of disability and its usefulness as a framework for researching later life.

The relevance of the disability movement

The starting point of the UK disability movement is its critique of the medical model of disability with its tendency to individualize or medicalize disability so that debate is reduced to a focus on the functional limitations of disabled individuals (Morris 1991; Oliver 1996). Instead, the movement favours the social model of disability based on the following distinctions:

> *Impairment*: lacking part or all of a limb, or having a defective limb, organism or mechanism of the body
>
> *Disability*: the disadvantage or restriction of activity caused by a contemporary social organization which takes no or little account of people who have impairments and this excludes them from the mainstream of social activities.
>
> (Oliver 1990: 11)

Whereas the medical world of disability is reducible to the individual, and stresses biological pathology, the social model locates the causes of disability squarely within society and social organization. Such a perspective defines disability as a political issue in which disabled people are offered the chance to join a social movement determined to win the right of disabled people to be full citizens of their society (Campbell and Oliver 1996).

In other words, many people have impairments but it is society which disables them through the denial of basic citizenship rights to

- work
- accommodation
- adequate income
- a full social life.

It is the social exclusion imposed by the lack of the above which oppresses disabled people rather than their impairments. Most health and welfare professionals stand accused of failing to campaign for the above rights because of their continued focus on the medical model, a focus encouraged by the fact that many of their jobs depend on the continued forced dependency of disabled people (Oliver 1990).

The impact of the disability movement upon social services, housing and to a lesser extent health has been profound. The disability movement has campaigned at the national and local levels, and has been very successful in encouraging the development of housing and support services which are, arguably, less stigmatizing than in the past and which encourage independent living. To take but two examples, the movement has played a pivotal role in the emergence of direct payment schemes by which disabled people buy in their own care workers (Hasler *et al.* 2000) and been a major participant (as Chapter 7 noted) in the whole debate about Lifetime Homes with the consequent amendment of the building regulations to improve access standards (Russell 1999).

To some extent older people with housing, health and social care needs have gained from this powerful challenge to old attitudes and assumptions. However, leading proponents of the disability movement acknowledge that it cannot claim to be a mass movement until older disabled people are much more centrally involved than they have been up to now (Campbell and Oliver 1996). However, as Means and Smith (1998a: 77) point out, 'this, of course, begs the question of whether older people whose experience of impairment may often not occur until later life are ever likely to identify in large numbers with the social model of disability and its political action implications'.

Another issue may be that older people are more likely to believe that their impairments and ill health do make a difference to their lives, and that the quality of their life will be affected by the quality of the support they receive from a range of health and welfare professionals. As such they might be inclined to agree with Morris's self-criticism that 'there is a tendency within the social model of disability to deny the experience of our own bodies, insisting that our physical differences and restrictions are entirely socially created' (Morris 1991: 10). Older people more than most need to come to terms with the restrictions of illness and the fear of dying, and hence may feel that some interpretations of the social model has its limitations.

Examples of older people's involvement in joint working

Older people may not be at the centre of the disability movement but there are growing examples of how they can be drawn into joint working as service users in a number of different ways. For example, older people forums are beginning to emerge and to demand a say in community care planning and other service developments (Carter and Nash 1993) while a number of authorities have experimented in the use of focus groups and/or teleconferencing in order to draw out the views of older service users (Wilson 1995), a trend which has been very much encouraged by the *Better Government for Older People* initiatives (2000). There have also been a number of interesting projects which have involved older people in the research process (Tozer and Thornton 1995). The need to develop feedback mechanisms from older people with dementia about the support they receive is now also recognized (Goldsmith 1996). Quite often, a common theme that comes through is that older people not only want to receive appropriate services but also to receive these from professionals who treat them with respect (Nocon and Qureshi 1996).

Perhaps one of the most interesting examples of involving older people comes from the work of Midgeley *et al.* (1997) who carried out extensive focus group interviews with older people, carers and professionals to identify the desired characteristics of an ideal housing and community care system. All three groups placed an emphasis upon the importance of independent living and linked to this decent housing was seen as a basic right which meant that new houses should be built with lifetime needs in mind. There was also a great emphasis upon choice, although respondents felt that housing should normally be provided to a mixed age group, with the 'special needs' of older people being met as part of this. Housing, health and social services professionals have less and less excuse for not involving older people in joint working.

Joined up thinking: the new mantra

This book has already made numerous references to 'joined up thinking' and 'joined up working' (see for example the discussion in Chapter 4 on public health), the importance of which has become almost a mantra for the present Labour government. Why is this? One of the driving agendas of this government is to create wealth and hence destroy poverty and deprivation through the creation of not only a full employment economy but also one based on a highly skilled and well-educated workforce. Through involvement in work and in the family, *all* members of society can be made to be full citizens who understand their rights and responsibilities, rather than there being a segment who are split off or socially excluded from the rest of society by their unemployment, poverty and fecklessness (see Powell 1999 for a fuller discussion of the social policies of the government). Flowing from this, the reason for the emphasis of the government upon 'Education, Education, Education' is clear as is the myriad of initiatives such as Health Action Zones and policy action teams that are designed to tackle geographical pockets of deprivation, poverty and health inequality. The emphasis is often upon young people or young single mothers and the aim is often to improve their educational skills and get them back in the labour market. But this is a government that recognizes the structural factors that generate deprivation and social exclusion rather than just emphasizing the need for individual decision making. Hence the need for a very wide range of professionals and agencies to work together at the structural and operational levels to defeat social exclusion.

One consequence of this emphasis upon citizenship, social exclusion and young people has been a marginalization of the needs of older people, especially in the single regeneration budget (SRB) and policy action team initiatives to tackle neighbourhood renewal. Riseborough (1999, 2000) in particular has been highly critical of this situation, pointing out 'that in those localities with high proportions of older people they are barely visible' (1999: 5). A preliminary analysis by Riseborough and colleagues of SRB/ Challenge bids for the Newcastle upon Tyne, Sandwell and Birmingham areas indicated that the contribution of older people was not recognized and that their needs and interests were only partially taken into account. Similarly, Fletcher (2000) presents findings on the links between regeneration and the housing aspects of community care. He showed that regeneration planning often fails to incorporate the housing, care and support needs of vulnerable people.

Despite this focus on young people in its social welfare programmes, the government has applied its joined up approach to the policy and practice of health and social care. The overall main driver may be social exclusion and young people, but the government believes that the same principle of joint working must be applied to tackling other major problems such as the high cost and ineffective nature of much health and social care available to older people. Both health (DoH 1997a) and social services (DoH 1998a) need to be modernized, and part of this modernization requires a greater emphasis upon working together. Thus, a key emphasis for the national priorities guidance for health and social care is the need to break down the barriers between services (DoH 1998d) while the discussion document, *Partnership in Action*, signalled a desire to remove blockages to joint working, especially with regard to the legality of pooled budgets (DoH 1998c). The initial circular on *Better Services for Vulnerable People* called for improved multidisciplinary assessment and rehabilitation services for older people (DoH 1997b) while the follow-up circular required local authorities and health authorities to establish joint investment programmes for older people by April 1999 (DoH 1998e). Finally, the Health Act 1999 has consolidated much of this thinking since it gives from April 2000 all principal local authorities and health authorities, NHS trusts and primary care trusts the power to pool budgets and resources, introduce lead commissioning and establish integral provision. Health and social services have been given a formal responsibility to work in partnership on the grounds that:

> People want and deserve the best public services . . . It is the responsibility of Government, local Government and the NHS to ensure that those justifiable expectations are met. People care about the quality of the services they get – not how they are delivered or who delivers them. We all need to make sure that service quality does not suffer because of artificial rigidities and barriers within and between service deliverers.
>
> (DoH/DETR 1999)

All of this seems very reasonable indeed especially since older people more than most have suffered from policy rigidities in the past as seen throughout this book and especially in Chapter 4. However, all this policy initiative around joined up thinking raises three crucial issues:

- How different are these policies from the joint working policies of the past?
- Are there any dangers in joint working?
- How difficult is joint working to deliver in practice?

Each of these questions will now be discussed in turn.

Old wine in new bottles?

It does need to be recognized that attempts to encourage joint working between health and social services, and sometimes with housing as well, has a very long history indeed. Webb (1991) has pointed out how exhortations to organizations, professionals and other producer interests to work together more closely and effectively litter the policy landscape and can be traced back at least as far as the Poor Law although the reality remains 'all too often a jumble of services fractionalised by professional, cultural and organizational boundaries and by tiers of government' (Webb 1991: 229).

Conservative governments of the late 1980s and 1990s seemed well aware of the need to encourage improved joint working. The Griffiths Report (1988) on community care, the White Paper on community care (DoH 1989) and the subsequent policy guidance (DoH 1990) are full of exhortations to joint working (see also Chapter 4). The lead role of social services in community care was meant to clarify working relationships with health; community care planning was to facilitate strategic working with a wide range of agencies including housing; and the care manager was to coordinate the care input of a wide range of providers.

It was a Conservative government and not the present Labour one who issued the guidance on establishing a strategic framework for housing and community care 'to help housing, social services and health authorities to establish joint strategies for housing and community care so that at a strategic level, the necessary co-ordination between housing, social services and health' can be achieved (DoH/DoE 1997; see also DoH 1999b). And it was the same government which commissioned the follow-up operational guidance for housing, health and social services on making partnerships work in community care (Means *et al.* 1997).

Yet it is unfair to claim that the policies of the Labour government on joined up working represent no more than 'old wine in new bottles'. Conservative governments may have stressed the importance of joint working but for them the driver for change was the discipline of the market in which

- market mechanisms should be used wherever possible, even if there cannot be a completely free market for services
- competition should be established between providers
- individualism and individual choice should take precedence over collective choices and planned provision
- state provision should be kept to a minimum, to encourage those who can afford it to opt out.

(based on Flynn 1989)

Although the Labour government is totally committed to the market economy and has a healthy respect for efficiency and effectiveness as demonstrated by its emphasis on Best Value (DETR 1998a), it does not believe in the hidden hand of the market to 'sort' health and welfare provision for such vulnerable groups as older people. Instead the emphasis is upon planning, priorities, targets and performance measurement (DoH 1999a). A key priority and target to be measured for both health and social services will be various aspects of working together, and this is a government that 'pays by results' so that financial penalties may well be incurred by those who fail to demonstrate that they are 'on message' with regard to joined up thinking. The commitment is much more than just a rehashing of old platitudes.

The dangers of joint working

So far the reader may well be of the view that joint working, especially as developed by the present government, is a wonderful thing that no right-thinking person could ever possibly disagree with or criticize under any circumstances. However, there are some real dangers in joint working. First, it can be used by governments to cover up inadequate funding. Perhaps the best example of this is housing investment itself. This book has profiled the lack of housing investment and consequent poor housing conditions that exist today and the impact of this on older people. Multi-agency renewal strategies and plans are fine. But at the end of the day these need to be backed up by adequate capital reinvestment. The present government would claim that it has reversed the public expenditure cuts of post-Conservative administrations. However, there is sometimes a suspicion that the same money is just being recycled around. Money is taken from one budget in order to fund a special initiative somewhere else.

Second, linked to this, it must always be remembered that joint working is not an end in itself. The performance measure needs to be the delivery of appropriate services to older people in need and not proof that staff from housing, health and social services are now meeting together on a regular basis. Indeed, the danger goes even deeper than that. Some forms of working together such as inter-agency assessment and referral protocols between housing and social services raise major issues about the rights of service users in terms of confidentiality and the passing on of information. As Means *et al.* (1997) explain, an element of information passing on is to be complimented: 'Service users and carers wish to see a wide spectrum of professionals working together to help obtain the right combination of services. This requires a willingness to share information' (Means *et al.* 1997: 7).

For example, such sharing of information is often crucial to the expedition of the housing allocation process. However, each agency needs 'to preserve confidentiality and supply information only on a need to know basis' (DoE/ DoH 1996). Drawing on *Building Bridges: A Guide to Arrangements for Inter-Agency Working for the Care and Protection of Severely Mentally Ill People* (DoH 1995), Means *et al.* (1997) argue that:

information passed on should be restricted to that in which the recipient has a legitimate interest; the recipient should not transmit it to a third party unless the latter is entitled to it or the patient either has explicitly consented or is aware that information needs to be passed on to enable care to be co-ordinated properly.

(Means *et al.* 1997: 53)

So what is the relevance of this to older people? We authors believe that vulnerable elders, and perhaps especially those with dementia, are highly likely to be treated in a way disrespectful of issues of confidentiality because everything is seen as being 'in their interests'. For example, although the enhanced care role of the sheltered housing warden (Hasler and Page 1998) is to be applauded, it is crucial that where possible the tenant is always con-sulted about any exchange of information between the warden, the health service and social services.

The final danger concerns the way in which a commitment to the 'common cause' of joint working can have the effect of stifling reasonable criticism and of undermining independent voices, especially in the voluntary sector which of course includes a very wide range of housing agencies including housing associations. Deakin (1995: 40) has talked of 'the perils of partnership' for this sector and perhaps especially for smaller associations since those 'with strong community connections have often acted as advocates and lobbyists on behalf of their users' (NFHA 1994). Joint working can be used to stifle dissent.

The challenge of joint working

A number of authors have outlined and discussed why joint working is easy to call for but extremely difficult to achieve in practice (Hudson 1987; Webb 1991; Hornby 1993; Owens *et al.* 1995; Huxham 1996). Their work suggests a number of common difficulties. The first is loss of autonomy. Joint working requires organizations and individuals to give up some autonomy to act inde-pendently, and they may lose some ability to set and control their own agenda and priorities. For example, housing associations, which are major providers of specialist housing for older people, have had to accept that new housing and care schemes may only be viable if control over nomination rights is ceded to social services. A second challenge is, beyond doubt, the cost of joint working. As Hudson (1987: 175) explains, 'working together requires agencies to invest scarce resources and energy in developing and maintaining relationships with other organizations when the potential returns are often unclear and intangible'. For example, small housing organizations like home improvement agencies, whose core client group is older people, may find it virtually impossible to engage with all the available joint working activ-ity that is ideally required of them in terms of both service delivery and contributing to strategic planning (Smart and Means 1997: 2).

The third challenge relates to the fact that professionals often hold negative stereotypes about each other and this can be especially true of housing and social services. So housing might think of social services in these terms:

There is the stereotyped image of the social worker as young and freshly qualified, straight from school via college, without any practical experience, who would be entirely subjective and idealistic about clients and will see all manner of handouts and special treatment for them without ever expecting them to stand on their own two feet.

> (quoted in Means and Smith 1998a: 194)

Social services might think of housing in the following way: 'I am not saying that they are a lot of heartless villains. I just think they are conditioned and they have little scope to do anything other than reach their targets in terms of rent arrears' (Clapham and Franklin 1994).

Our own teaching experiences with housing and social work students suggest that elements of such stereotypes still exist, and it is certainly true that the more entrenched the stereotypes, the harder it will be to develop joint working.

Another challenge is the existence of cultural differences both between professionals and between agencies. Assumptions about how to understand and respond to need may be different, and each profession or type of agency may have its own jargon. This links to another issue which relates to disagreements about roles and responsibilities which has been a striking feature of the often poor relationship between health authorities/trusts and social services especially over continuing care responsibilities for older people (Means and Smith 1998a, 1998b). But it is also an issue with regard to roles and responsibilities towards tenants with support needs including older people. Housing often feel dumped upon as a result of what is perceived as the irresponsible behaviour of health and social services as exemplified by this quote from a sheltered housing warden with three residents with diagnosed dementia: 'Again, twit syndrome, you're there and they think that's okay. They can just send (the old person) and you'll catch the lot because don't forget as soon as they put one step over their own threshold they're your problem' (Langan and Means, 1995).

Health and social care professionals involved in the case would probably refer to their large caseloads but also query whether the warden had ever made a clear enquiry of them to visit and reassess. Overall the message with regard to joint working is that it is often undermined by misunderstandings:

> professionals often have only limited knowledge about other professional groups or other organizations with which they wish to liaise and work with. They simply misunderstand the priorities, organizational structures, cultures and working practices of potential partners, and how this relates to very real statutory differences.
>
> (Means *et al.* 1997: 8)

This is certainly the case in housing, health and social services. Arblaster *et al.* (1996) carried out a national postal survey combined with three case studies on inter-agency working and found an overall failure to communicate, caused partly by a lack of conceptual understanding about the overall functions of each other and partly by a lack of awareness of what each did in practice on a day-to-day basis.

So how can we overcome these problems? Hudson (1987) points out that there are only three main strategies for encouraging reluctant agencies to work together. As Means and Smith (1998a: 141) explain, these are coopera-tive strategies (based on mutual agreements), incentive strategies (based on 'bribes' to encourage joint working) and authoritative strategies (agencies are instructed to 'work together'). As we saw earlier in this chapter, the tendency of central government is increasingly to use a mixture of authori-tative and incentive strategies with health and social services, backed up the presentation of evidence from the Audit Commission (1997) and other research to demonstrate that joint working is cost effective and hence worth the opportunity cost. However, housing is more often left on the side-lines of these developments as being a desirable rather than essential partner.

At the locality level and at the operational level, strategies for joint working are much more likely to be based upon a mixture of cooperation and low-level incentives (such as free places on training courses, recognition of support for a neighbourhood network in one's workload, and so on). Under these circum-stances, it is crucial for those keen to stimulate and support joint working across housing, health and social services to

- obtain backing from senior managers
- identify objectives and real gains for all participants (joint initiatives which only meet the objectives of the instigator are almost certain to fail)
- map the organizational structures, priorities and key actors of all the participating agencies
- build up trust so that collaborative partners work in the first instance on modest tasks with modest objectives, especially when there has been a past history of conflict and distrust. Success from such ventures creates the platform from which to go to more challenging initiatives in the future.

(based on Webb 1991)

The overall message is perhaps that joint working is difficult but can be made to work and that an understanding of other professions and agencies is a crucial starting point.

Making partnerships work in community care (the content)

So what does all of this mean for hard-pressed housing, health and social services staff? As already indicated, *Making Partnerships Work in Community Care: A Guide for Practitioners in Housing, Health and Social Services* (Means *et al.* 1997) has the status of official practice guidance from both the Department of Health and the DETR. Its whole thrust is to offer support for busy practi-tioners to make joint working happen on the ground by looking at the follow-ing issues, all of them highly relevant to older people's interests:

- the challenge of joint working
- mapping your locality

- assessment and care management
- home adaptation and home improvement
- housing agencies and primary health-care teams
- hospital admission and discharge.

Running through the workbook is the encouragement for professionals to get to know how other professionals and other agencies are organized in their localities. For example, housing professionals are asked if they know the explicit priorities used to decide who qualifies for a care package by social services. An example is given of an authority in which the priorities for older people are as follows:

- Priority 1 To provide appropriate community-based services in order to reduce the requirement for some older people (including those with carers) with complex needs to enter residential or nursing home care on a long-term basis.
- Priority 2 To support carers who themselves may need support to enable them to continue caring.
- Priority 3 To enhance the quality of life of carers and users.

However, the priority guidance also informed care managers that 'within existing budgets, it is not expected that it will be possible to purchase services to help people who fall in the Priority 3 categories' (Means *et al.* 1997: 21). A major source of tension between operational staff from housing and social services can be a lack of understanding of the systems for prioritizing those in greatest need which exist in social services. It is thus crucial that housing professionals identify the priority systems used by their local social services department.

Health and social services professionals equally need to develop their knowledge and understanding of the organization of housing within their localities. Finally, it is crucial that both housing and social services also map the complex new arrangements for primary care (see Chapter 4) in their localities. The overall assumption is that mapping localities in this kind of way will greatly increase the effectiveness of joint working by providing a clear picture of other key agencies.

Linked to this, there is also a need for much greater clarity about the respective roles of housing, social services and health. For example in terms of why social services might need to involve housing, it is possible to identify three broad areas. First, the care manager may not be sure of their client's housing needs and hence wishes to access a specialist housing needs assessment around a wide range of issues. These include damp in the house, tenancy rights, entitlement to a home improvement grant, whether they are homeless as defined by housing legislation or about whether their housing is inappropriate. Allen *et al.*'s (1998) work on assessing housing needs in community care suggests that the housing needs of older people are inadequately picked up via community care assessments. Second, the care manager might wish to access housing or housing services for their client (for example a council house, a housing association property, a housing with support scheme, or a home adaptation.) Third, the care manager may need to work with the housing professional to address issues of, for example, rent arrears, housing disrepair and maintenance or conflict with neighbours.

In a similar way, housing might need to bring in social services for a range of reasons. First, the housing professional may not be sure of the care and support needs of their client and hence wish to access a specialist community care assessment. Second, the housing professional may wish to access services provided or funded by social services such as home care, respite care or a place in a residential or nursing home. Finally, the housing professional may need to work with the care manager to sort out the existing care package of a tenant, to address issues relating to the distressing behaviour of neighbours known to social services or to assess whether the housing situation of a tenant is exacerbating social care needs.

From this perspective, it is essential to clarify the basic knowledge about housing that should be held by social services staff and the basic knowledge about community care that is needed by housing staff. The judgement of the workbook is that housing staff need to have the following skills and knowledge:

- awareness of how social services and health are organized locally, what their priorities are and what they might realistically be likely to provide
- knowledge of how to make appropriate referrals to health and social services, including information required by social services
- knowledge of signs of possible dementia and when to seek further advice
- ability to recognize possible signs of crisis and vulnerability
- alternative sources of help and advice (advocacy groups, organizations of service users/disabled people, specialist voluntary agencies, and so on)
- a commitment to work in partnership with the tenant, housing applicant or their advocate.

It is recognized that housing staff cannot demand that health and social services provide services. However, they can encourage a specialist assessment to be made where they have concerns about a client or tenant.

In a similar way, the workbook identifies the skills and knowledge required of social services staff about housing. These are seen as including:

- awareness of how housing is organized locally, what their priorities are and what housing agencies might realistically be likely to provide (NB: housing authorities must provide free copies of a summary of their housing allocations schemes)
- this awareness to include an understanding of both options for homeless people and vulnerable tenants, together with options for those seeking advice on home improvement and/or adaptation
- knowledge of how to make appropriate referrals to housing agencies; knowledge of how to respond appropriately to referrals from housing agencies
- awareness of alternative sources of help and advice (advocacy groups, organizations of service users/disabled people, specialist voluntary agencies, and so on)
- commitment to work in partnership with service users and their advocates.

It is emphasized that social services staff cannot demand a response from housing agencies but they can encourage a (re)assessment to be made where they have concerns about their client's housing situation.

The argument of the workbook is that from such an agreed base, staff from housing and social services will become much more effective and knowledgeable about how to refer service users on for more specialist assessment and support. One of the biggest challenges is to develop an equivalent level of clarity in joint working between housing and primary care.

Making partnerships work in community care (the process)

The workbook is about making partnerships work in community care. Interestingly, it was produced only as a result of a major piece of joint working which spanned numerous stakeholders. The workbook had to be acceptable to two government departments which had little history of effective joint working around housing, health and community care issues. Even within each department, a number of sections/divisions had a right to comment on different draft modules of the workshop according to whether the focus was home improvement/adaptation, hospital discharge, primary care or whatever. The steering group for the project contained a wide range of other key stakeholders including the NHS Executive, the Housing Corporation, the National Users and Carers Group and the local authority associations. The authors were also required to work with a practitioner panel of 24 people, all with their own views about everything from the overall style of the workbook through to issues of detailed content. The authors also worked closely with two individual service user consultants and a group of older people from a service users' network. Finally the work had to be cleared by ministers in a situation where the content of the workbook had been produced under a Conservative government but was to be published under a Labour government about to make radical changes in many aspects of health and social care policy.

The challenges to successful completion were considerable. For example, the change in government very close to publication required considerable redrafting and the production of a post-publication policy update. On one occasion a fax was received requesting that all references to 'private sector initiatives' should be amended to read 'public private partnerships'. However, more significantly, there were strikingly different views between the Department of Health and the DETR about aspects of the workbook. Sometimes, there were simple questions of favoured terminology with the DETR still comfortable with the term 'special needs', which had been largely rejected by the Department of Health and, of course, completely rejected by all those commenting from a service user perspective.

Perhaps the most fascinating difference occurred over the issue of confidentiality (and how to protect it) in the context of improved joint working between health and social services. The view of the DETR tended to be that housing officers were often put at risk from people with mental health problems as a result of the failure (or the refusal) of social services to share information about their clients. The view of the authors, which was broadly supported by the Department of Health, was that joint working must not be used as an excuse to pass on vast amounts of (probably irrelevant) information about clients and to do this in a way which does not seek their permission for this to happen.

The first draft had a suggested 'good practice' form which generated a tick and the comment 'excellent' from the Department of Health but a cross and the comment 'it must not appear' from the DETR. In the end, the detailed talking through of the issue plus excellent guidance from one of the service user consultants enabled a way forward to be found and this was based upon two components. First, it was agreed that the workbook needed to draw upon existing government backed guidance. Thus, the workbook quotes the *Code of Guidance in Parts VI and VII of the Housing Act 1996*:

> There may be occasions . . . where the sharing of such information is sensible and can expedite the allocation process . . . although authorities will wish to preserve confidentiality and supply information only on a 'need to know' basis.
>
> (DoE/DoH 1996: 2)

This was supported by the more detailed good practice suggestions from the government offered in *Building Bridges* (DoH 1995) from which it was possible to develop a 'good practice' checklist for the workbook (see Table 8.2). The second component of the workbook process was to encourage the DETR to think in terms of risk assessment. It was successfully argued that the mass passing on of confidential information to housing offices about vast numbers of social services clients not only would be unethical but also would be counter-productive. Housing would become overloaded with such information and this would reduce the capacity of identifying the very small number who were 'at risk', in terms of their own well-being or their capacity to harm others.

It is interesting to reflect upon why the workbook was successfully completed despite the range of difficulties faced and how this relates to the

Table 8.2   'Need to know' good practice checklist

1 Have you agreed with the service user or their advocate the *details* of what information may be passed on?
2 Have you been clear and precise on why you are passing information over? (What purpose is it meeting?)
3 Have you been clear about who is to receive the information and the extent to which others will have access to the information once passed over?
4 Have you involved individuals and their advocates when passing on the required information? (Don't assume that the professional always has to do this.)
5 Have you been honest to the service user or their advocate if you feel required to pass certain information over irrespective of their agreement (perhaps because of previous offences)?
6 Have you sought flexible solutions which enable service users to have their needs met according to their own preferences?

Source: Means *et al.* 1997: 54

literature reviewed earlier in the chapter. The workbook certainly gained from having a number of champions. The lead officers from both the Department of Health and the DETR were committed to the workbook and hence willing to invest in time to talk through differences and disagreements. The authors were also passionate about the workbook and hence were willing to invest time in problem solving over and above formal contractual obligations.

There was a high level of trust among key players. The lead officers had worked together on the preceding housing and community care circular (DoH/DoE 1997) while the senior author of the workbook had liaised with the Department of Health lead officer on two previous projects. All of this suggests the existence of a collaborative approach to making a success of joint working. However, the workbook was also something that had been commissioned and local authorities (and others) had been told to expect. Neither the commissioned authors nor the two government departments could afford to be seen as failing to do this. As such these were very strong incentives for success, which was close to what Hudson (1987) calls an authoritative strategy in which agencies are ordered to work together.

All of this enabled those closely associated with the workbook to overcome the usual misunderstandings, negative stereotypes, worries about loss of autonomy, cultural differences and conflicts over roles and responsibilities which so often characterize complex attempts at working together. However, it can be argued that the workbook also illustrated two of the great potential weaknesses of a heavy policy and practice reliance on joint working. First, its production placed a high opportunity cost upon key players in terms of meetings and generally working through problems. Second, some practitioner panel members remained concerned that it was being offered as a substitute for the adequate resourcing of services.

These weaknesses demand some reflections on the impact of the workbook and how this relates to the cost of its production. Both the Department of Health and the DETR proved willing to fund regional dissemination workshops in 1998 and 1999. These were organized in terms of trying to persuade key organizations in localities to come as cross-agency teams so that they could work together on 'real' issues on the day of the workshop. Each workshop was co-hosted by the regional offices of the Government Office, the NHS Executive and the Social Services Inspectorate. The impact of these workshops was never followed up but one suspects that for many they became just one more event. Aspirations by the authors to use the workbook as an action research tool with enthusiastic localities were never pursued. Although mentioned in the White Paper on *Modernising Social Services* (DoH 1998a), one suspects that the workbook has become 'yesterday's news' despite the very significant investment made in it. We hope that the workbook has made a significant contribution in some localities to fostering a joined up solution approach to working with older people across housing, health and social services. However, elsewhere one suspects that many of the old rigidities and resource limitations remain despite the positive emphasis on change and modernization propounded by the present government.

Conclusion

This chapter has argued that the present emphasis of the Labour government upon joint working across housing, health and social services shows a recognition of the need for professionals to focus upon the needs of older people rather than the temptation to defend narrow organizational self-interest. It has also looked at some of the many obstacles to effective joint working and gone on to illustrate how two of the authors of this book (Means and Heywood) were involved in guidance which aimed to overcome at least some of these problems on the ground (Means *et al.* 1997).

The discussion of the production of the workbook has illustrated just how difficult it can be to make real progress and gave a warning that joint working can so often be a mechanism for deflecting attention away from inadequate resourcing. However, it must be remembered that service users want a coherent response to their needs from a wide range of agencies and this requires housing, health and social services professionals not only to improve their general skills at joint working but also to develop their confidence to find ways of involving older people in this process. We hope that the workbook has made a small contribution to achieving this.

9

Conclusions

The subject 'housing and older people' has often been viewed as a set of technical problems. It has been confined to a small area within specialized housing or care and hence has largely ignored the 90 per cent of the older population who do not live in such provision. As a subject area within housing studies it has been largely marginalized, despite the efforts of various researchers including, at times, the three of us. Nor has it any real substantive place in social gerontology although environment is usually recognized as one of the components of quality of life. Here, we take up the challenge that we set ourselves at the beginning of the book which was to rethink the place of housing and home in later life. We said that there was largely a vacuum where policies existed and such policies that did exist tended to be both ageist and located within a medical model of disability.

Immediately a very real problem comes up. Are we not undermining this book's central message if we propose a set of housing policies tailor made to later life? We have argued in various places (in Chapters 1 and 2 in particular) that old people are not a race apart. There is a worry that distinct housing policies such as the innovative forms of communal living (discussed in Chapter 7) and Care and Repair or Staying Put projects (discussed in Chapter 6) may deepen the tendency to segregate and discriminate on the grounds of old age. It is a problem, of course, that many others have worked with. Jamieson *et al.* (1997) come down on the side of emphasizing the distinct characteristics of later life in order to develop a critique of how older people are discriminated against. However, they argue for a focus on the life course and adult life rather than on older people in order to overcome the problems of age based definitions. Bernard and Phillips (2000) are also against a focus on old age as such but argue for an integrated social policy which addresses the broad needs of an ageing society:

Within an intergenerational life course perspective, ageing therefore seems to us to have more of a potential than a focus on old age or old people . . . it begins to move us away from the idea that there is a separate and distinct group we can all clearly identify as 'old'. In this context we would also argue for the need to rid ourselves of the divisiveness of the increasingly prevalent and uncritical use of the terms 'third' and 'fourth' age.

(Bernard and Phillips 2000: 44)

In this chapter we want largely to embrace the position held by Jamieson *et al.* (1997). At this point in social gerontology's development we want to focus on the distinct characteristics of later life in order to draw attention to and do something constructive about the policy vacuum which the book has revealed. Such a position accords with the critical gerontological paradigm that we favoured in Chapter 2. However, *at the same time* we want to endorse the integrated social policy approach advocated by Bernard and Phillips (2000). We argue that housing is central to an integrated social policy. Housing policy, indeed, is fundamental to the process of ageing. Housing and home are the ideal vehicles for moving to a more inclusive view of ageing, one that begins at youth and continues until death. Housing is a fundamental right. Bad housing policies can wreak havoc with people's lives, their health and their life chances. But, equally, good housing policies may be able to reverse these trends. The policy of Lifetime Homes (discussed in Chapter 6) is a very clear example. Were domestic environments more adequately built for the needs of the majority and not just for a super race of modal height, weight and age, special treatment of older and disabled people through the delivery of adaptations would be less necessary. Good quality housing policies for all promote social inclusion. The poor health of older people is partly a consequence of years of failure in British housing policy and inadequate housing for young people today is laying a sure path to more ill health and social need when they become the older people of the future.

Current policies

It is important now to summarize the critique of current policies which have been presented in this book. One of the aims of the introductory chapter was to show how important history is in understanding current policies. The historical analysis presented showed that over the past hundred years or so older people's housing careers were shaped by, primarily, social and economic policies. The analysis also noted changes and continuities. As far as discontinuities with the past are concerned, the increase in numbers of older people living alone and tenure change must surely be the most important. Both these social indicators have enormous policy implications. Tenure change in favour of owner occupation has contributed to housing becoming a privatized, hidden away, issue and as such, highly convenient for governments. However, the rise in home-ownership has worked to the advantage of some older people. A further change is that laissez-faire policies gave way to the general acceptance that the imperfections of the market have to be modified through welfare provision. Some factors remained constant throughout the twentieth century – namely the vast majority of older people lived as independent householders in ordinary housing with support coming from mainly the family, not the state. Moreover, throughout the century, the state support people that did get in their own homes was inadequate.

The historical themes of the opening chapter were taken up in Chapter 2 and subsequent chapters. The paternalism and fear of creating dependency through the provision of welfare, inspired by Octavia Hill and the Charity Organization Society, has not disappeared. For example, the development of sheltered housing was justified in terms of the 'special' support that older people wanted. Such housing policies paper over the cracks and can divert structured inequalities in later life into the culture of blame. Even with the Staying Put policies of the 1980s, which we welcome because they can make it easier for people to remain in their own homes, the underlying 'discourse' is in terms of individualizing and pathologizing – 'Older people need help with patching up their homes because they lack sufficient energy and expertise to tackle the difficult task of arranging and funding home improvement'.

Chapter 2 also subjected contemporary housing policy to some theoretical analysis borrowing from a number of different disciplines. A further theme was that of the strong links between theories of later life and theories of disability. The empirical evidence is never so clear as with housing. The social model of disability has been unpopular with some students of later life because it associates old age with impairment, an association many older people would reject. However, impairment is statistically correlated with age. It is certainly true that many older people themselves normalize their impairments by simply getting on with life but such behaviour is highly convenient to penny pinching governments who can thus continue not to respond to or alleviate pain and discomfort which are made worse by unsuitable and poor quality housing. Discrimination against older people is rife within the NHS and every other part of the social welfare system. Governments can continue to ignore the unhealthy effects of non-barrier-free disabling housing. Some of the concepts from within disability studies do not translate easily into the study of later life nor vice versa but politically the social model of disability could be an effective mechanism for combating the powerful and often covert ageism which so heavily permeates housing and social policies directed at older people. The model could also come into service provision (as Chapter 6 implied) as a basis for improving the delivery of adaptation services. Also (as Chapter 8 noted), it is a powerful vehicle for improving older people's involvement in joint working.

The discourse of the social model of disability can question an equally influential discourse, namely that of 'independent living'. The latter has been particularly successful at misleading its audience into believing that there has been a major sea change in the way older people are viewed and that housing is a major plank within independent living policies. Independent living has now become the new mantra and, like motherhood and apple pie, it is almost impossible to contest. Housing is seen as a central component of independent living. Chapter 4 charted the evolution of the turnabout in housing's fortunes as far as community care is concerned. The integration of housing with community care is to be truly welcomed in the sense that it has brought short-term improvement to older people. It means, for example, that resources may be put into providing a stair-lift so that a person can avoid a move to an institution. However, the discourse is dangerous because it conceals a continued negative approach to older people. Independent living as a discourse often has less to do with genuine principles of empowerment, normalization and of choice and control and very much more to do with saving the state money and re-establishing people's dependency on their relatives, or, to use community care parlance, informal carers. Good housing is crucial to the quality of life of older people but so often it has been embraced as part of the community care 'project', that is, reducing reliance on residential care. Allen (1997) has argued that housing's role in community care is very narrowly construed:

> the housing role in community care is not a symbolic representation of political commitment to the conceptual principles cited above (*i.e. empowerment, normalization, social role valorization, independent living, etc*) or even a policy objective. Conversely housing forms the central means of achieving other policy objectives. The housing role is therefore salient to the policy framework for its 'function' of integrating disabled people into communities where ideologically and economically significant networks of informal care can be tapped, thus enabling disabled people to attain independence from state provision . . . Housing is merely important for its 'functional' importance (i.e. as a means) and not its political importance (i.e. as an end) to the policy framework.
>
> (Allen 1997: 96, added emphasis)

For the purposes of our argument in this book, for disabled people in the above quotation we would ask you to substitute older people. Home is where most people want to be; they quite unsurprisingly fear residential care and may dislike the idea of sheltered housing but the processes of institutionalization can be as pervasive 'at home' as well 'as in a home' (Baldwin *et al.* 1993; Reed and Payton 1996). Ill health and immobility institutionalize older people and the process of assessment and subsequent care delivery from bureaucratic organizations can so often exacerbate an older person's dependent status wherever they are living.

The strong message coming from policy statements is that older people wish to stay in their *own* homes. This is the case with the majority of older people but the independent living discourse deliberately obfuscates. *Own* home is intended to mean *existing* home, not a suitable home that affords some satisfaction to the person living there. As Chapter 5 and other chapters of this book have noted, research studies often conclude there are older people who do wish move from their unsuitable home to a better home but face considerable obstacles or constraints.

Linked to the concept of independent living is the relatively recent discouragement in housing policy of special needs or supported housing. This is now manifested in a whole number of initiatives including most recently the *Supporting People* proposals discussed in several chapters of this book (DSS 1998b). The avowed purpose of *Supporting People* is to uncouple accommodation from support and find ways of supporting people in their own homes rather than in 'schemes'. Throughout the book we have shown ourselves to be strongly in support of anti-special-needs arguments. However, as with independent living, we have pointed out the power of these arguments when deployed by governments to mislead. It is highly convenient for policy makers, facing all the usual problems thrown up in the wake of globalization and the new postmodern world, to argue against 'provision' and 'schemes' saying they are segregationalist. It is also convenient for them to argue that everyone wants to live in their *existing* homes. Reducing public expenditure is often the imperative, not meeting the social and collective needs of some older people. Older people do not seem to want to live in special needs schemes designated as such and called all sorts of things like close care, sheltered housing, very sheltered housing, assisted living and so on. What some, however, want is to live with others of a similar age with the aim of achieving, possibly, a better quality of life. They want to choose when to move. In the words of the Dutch co-housing resident referred to in Chapter 7: 'It is important to move to a place you choose before other people move you to a place they choose'. It is ironic also that governments are not against older people moving from their existing homes when those homes are family homes in the social rented sector. Here the language is different; housing benefit must be reduced or under-occupation minimized.

The final point in the independent living/anti-special-needs housing debate concerns definitions. Independent living is a difficult and complex concept and yet, so often, it is trivialized to mean simply the opposite of dependent living, which in turn is something that is largely reviled. We have produced much evidence in this book to suggest that ideas of housing providers about independent living and those of older people are not always going to line up. For example independence may represent the ability to demand a service which one is paying for from a helper as an alternative to depending on the vagaries of complicated and possibly emotionally laden family care. Independence is so often contrasted with dependency. The former is good and the latter bad. But why should being dependent on others be denigrated? For us, the key issue is not whether housing and social policies contribute to independence but whether they improve quality of life.

We now turn to rather more specific examples of ageist and unhelpful policies which have been discussed throughout the book. Chapter 3 made the point that the main reason why housing is not seen as central to the later life agenda is that post-war governments have been so successful at privatizing housing both literally and as an issue. The aim of the chapter was to give very concrete examples of dissonance between what older people would like to get from housing policy and the current response from national and local government. Housing need has been very narrowly defined in the interests of achieving the best use of resources. Help with housework, with gardening, with decorating and with odd jobs are all desired activities and crucial to successful 'independent living' but, so often, argued over by different agencies and, so often, left undone. The deployment of scarce social housing resources, for example, has meant that under-occupation is a big worry for policy makers and older people's desire for space goes unheeded. Requirements for a decent amount of space are ridden over roughshod through attempts to restrict housing benefit. The root and branch reform of the latter which is expected in the not too distant future promises no joy for older people unless policies of reducing bricks and mortar subsidy are drastically reformed. Allocation policies are also very narrowly drawn and repair and improvement strategies, although they do try to recognize the particular interests of older people, are very underfunded. Chapter 3 also continued the themes of Chapters 1 and 2. It showed that governments are skilled at deception and words are given a twist. For example, in submission to the Royal Commission, civil servants maintained that older people were receiving better services. Although this may be true of some of those presently receiving services, the reality is that fewer people than in the past have been given anything. It could, therefore, be argued that the overall situation for older people is worse. Another theme which the chapter was concerned with is paternalism, control and assessment. Older people's voices are so often ignored. Good practice example such as the Fife user panels and local authorities like Cornwall where assessment has been abandoned are few and far between. *Supporting People* (DSS 1998b) seemed like a new beginning. It promised a radical policy and funding framework for providing low-level, preventive support services to people wherever they live, for example to older people owning their own housing as well as to sheltered housing tenants. However, as the detail on its implementation unfolds it seems more and more that assessment by somebody other than the older person will continue, as will the old monolithic system of block grant which currently characterizes supported housing.

In Chapter 4 the connections between health and housing received a thorough airing. Although there is now a recognition in public health policies of the contribution of housing to health, this has not been thought about in any detail in the context of the health and welfare of older people. The chapter highlighted the important and, so often, neglected links between mental health and housing. The policy discussions of Chapter 4 connect up to the empirical research reported in Chapter 8. Chapter 8 takes further the exploration of the links between housing and community care in the context of an exposition on the importance of joint working. Joined up thinking in local decision making is demanded by a government that continues to govern in a non-joined-up way at the centre. Joint working can be a snare and a delusion in just the same way as independent living and the attack on special needs thinking. It can so often be a rationale for reducing the total amount of resources available. But older and disabled people do want good quality joined up working because they want a coordinated response from health and welfare professionals.

Emerging from both Chapters 4 and 8 is the issue of boundaries. This government that is so concerned about joined up thinking is obsessed with separating out housing, health and social care so that budgets can be separately charged. However, people's lives are not fragmented in this way; people require a seamless service. Chapter 7 also discussed boundaries. In addition the chapter concluded that to live in any communal setting in Britain is seen as something which is rather negative and which only has to happen sometimes when it is uneconomic to support and care for people in their own homes. What we have in Britain now is two systems of provision existing side by side, one residential care and the other the various forms of sheltered housing. Their boundaries have blurred in terms of their purpose and aims and in who they accommodate but structurally they are distinct and produce different outcomes. Residential care is subject to regulation and inspection. A blanket fee is charged for accommodation, living expenses and care which allows for no flexibility. Residents are pauperized in terms of very low disposable incomes. Sheltered housing is not registered. Residents have housing rights and their 'own front doors' and are eligible for housing benefit and related benefits.

Chapter 5 looked at moving and reiterated the finding that older people move far less often than the younger population. This residential stability has in the past been generally explained in terms of individual pathology, in terms often of older people lacking energy with which to make the necessary organizational arrangements. The chapter shows that more needs to be understood about moving and not moving in later life. It puts forward a methodology that, by taking a holistic view of people's housing needs, shows why supposedly suitable options will so often be unacceptable. It details the lack of options and steady decline in housing investment and hence in the opportunities to move during the 1980s and 1990s. More needs to be understood about tenure switch and the release of housing wealth when trading down is achieved.

Chapter 6 showed that some of the best policies for older people lie in renovation, adaptation and new build. The policies have been good, they have been sensitive and they can, in theory, make a real difference to people's lives. But the chapter concluded that so often theory does not convert into reality because of two factors, severe underfunding and negative and discriminatory attitudes to older people on the part of those who implement policies. The chapter also noted the enormous importance of good design to people's lives.

A new start for housing policy

These, then, are the main difficulties with current policies. We now need to consider what changes can be made and the extent to which these changes can be implemented. In his exposition on later life at the end of the twentieth century Phillipson (1998) is gloomy. Later life in the context of globalization is characterized by risk and uncertainty and still associated with major inequalities. Phillipson and others, for example Bernard and Phillips (2000), also feel that the new consumerism does not give older people any real rights or power. During the late 1980s and 1990s self-provisioning became more and more commonplace and only those with very few financial resources of their own received state subsidies for housing and care services. Yet, although the language is now one of consumers and choice, even those who have to pay for themselves are still treated in paternalistic and ageist ways.

However, there do seem to be some grounds for being rather less than pessimistic about the opportunities for promoting positive change. First, the amount of money available for housing investment for 2000–2001 has increased for the first time in many years. Second, the language has changed. Increasingly, older people are being described as 'citizens' and 'empowerment' is a word that rolls off the tongue. Although at the moment this is no more than just a change in the discourse, it is helpful and could lead to a change of mind set. Third, a key historical change which has largely gone unremarked by social gerontologists is the massive tenure change that has gone on. This has powerful social, political and economic implications. Researchers such as Hancock (2000) have painstakingly mapped the level of housing equity held by an ever increasing proportion of the older population. Although, as we have noted at various points in this book, there have been unrealistic expectations of this resource, nevertheless for some people home-ownership and the wealth attached gives them leverage and rather more possibilities in terms of housing and care options. Again, we know surprisingly little about older people's attitudes to their housing wealth and their views about preserving it for future generations. As Chapter 5 showed, researchers looking at mobility and later life have largely focused on issues to do with negative status passages and the inevitable difficulties of moving when coping in the existing home is difficult. Although we know there is widespread resentment on the part of many older people about having to sell houses to pay for residential care, trading down for *some* older people can and does release substantial sums. They may, thus, be able to act much more like consumers than the popular image of later life supposes.

Nor is acting like a consumer necessarily confined to that minority of the ageing population with expensive houses to trade. With marketization has come the expectation that older people should behave like consumers but researchers have largely been uninterested in examining whether older people are beginning to respond to these trends. Some of the paradigms of later life which were discussed in Chapter 2 have not been interested in 'agency'. Although many older people have insubstantial financial resources they are not passive beings in the face of huge societal developments. Evidence from the studies reported on in Chapter 7, for example, suggest they can take on the consumer role thrust upon them. A very good example lies in the customary distinction between self-payers and publicly funded residents of care homes. Both groups felt they were paying for the care delivered to them. The local authority funded residents had to give up all their income minus a few pounds a week which can be retained as 'personal allowance' or 'pocket money'. They appeared to feel as entitled as the self-payers to be critical of service delivery.

In pulling together the ideas and information covered in the book we propose change at several levels and in several areas. Below we deal with

- new approaches to research
- a new mind set
- involvement of older people
- an integrated social policy approach
- making a reality of the preventive agenda
- dealing with boundary issues
- redefining joint working
- redefining housing need.

New approaches to research

What is needed is more research within ageing studies or social gerontology on housing and home and more research within housing studies on later life. We need to know far more than we do at the moment about the relationship between home and self-identity. The plea we make here is for far more notice to be taken of housing and home factors in ageing studies. As Chapters 2 and 5 have shown, our understanding of the meaning of home is very restricted. For example, remarkably little is known about tenure and its impact on the life course. We also want to ask for a different style of research than that often carried out. The key difficulty is that the vast majority of research into old age is conducted by 'not old' researchers. So often assumptions are made which are not always valid. Although a wide variety of methodologies should be employed, the current bias towards measurement and structured approaches could be tilted slightly in the favour of a range of qualitative techniques which involve listening to older people's accounts. Currently a strong user perspective can often be missing. Researchers can be no different from policy makers and providers. Messages from older people go unheard.

A new mind set

Oversimplifying, there are two reasons why the issue of housing and older people is neglected: one is lack of funding and the other is attitudinal. The two, however, are inextricably linked. What is needed are mechanisms which can move the new talk of citizenship and empowerment beyond discourse into a new type of service delivery. This cannot just be done through training courses targeted to a series of different professionals but has to be tackled at many different levels. The fear, of course, is that a move from the prevailing medical model with its focus on activities of daily living assessment and care management will lead to the unleashing of demands which, in a resource constrained world, cannot possibly be met. The existing evidence, however, points the other way. For example, employing a social model of disability approach to the allocation of housing to disabled people has been found to lead to more cost-effective deployment of resources (Shaw 1999). So often adaptations for example, are not used because they were not wanted. Moreover, the example of Cornwall, described in Chapter 3, where community care assessments gave way to giving people what they asked for shows that overall costs can be reduced. The most effective method, perhaps of arriving at a new mind set which would influence researchers, policy makers and practitioners alike, is to involve older people in the policy and practice process.

Involvement of older people

User participation is so much easier to exhort than to achieve, yet in the area of service delivery to older people it is long overdue. It needs to be championed in so many different ways; for example older people as researchers; older people as experts on the design of living environments (whether they are houses, public buildings, residential care homes or sheltered housing); older people as self-assessors when it comes to service provision and so on. As far as policy developments are concerned, older people have not been adequately involved or consulted. There are a spate of initiatives currently but these are mainly provider inspired and are usually driven by funding and policy factors. We have very little idea what older people's views are of different living arrangements and different housing and support models. For example, in the focus groups the research commissioned by the Royal Commission conducted a great deal of confusion emerged as to the difference between sheltered housing and residential care. There are examples of user involvement. The *Better Government for Older People* initiatives discussed earlier are one and so are the Fife user panels. However, they need to be followed up by other examples where user consultation is succeeded by action which leads, as far as the participants are concerned, to positive change. Best Value is a further example where, in theory, users are consulted. Here the worry always is that consultation is tokenistic. Finally, there are interesting examples of housing-led user initiative, non-age specific, such as tenant participation compacts which give council tenants a real say in the management of their homes.

An integrated social policy approach

Bernard and Phillips (2000) want to move away from a narrow conceptualization of social policy of ageing towards an intergenerational approach. Housing and home, or (as these authors have it) the 'spatial dimension of life', are ideal settings. Put simply, well-funded broad-based housing policies for all do away with the need to focus on the distinct characteristics of old age. We have already put forward Lifetime Homes as good example but there are others. One example lies in urban regeneration. As a Debate of the Age Millennium Paper (Russell 1999) says, the concept of the balanced community is a way of solving some of the problems with the built environment in which we currently live. What we therefore propose is housing policies which promote balanced communities. The latter are made up of a mixture of people in terms of class, income age, ethnicity and household type and provide a range of services, homes, schools, employment and transport, all easily accessible to their residents They also tend to exhibit high levels of attachment to and participation in community life, mutual support and skills sharing.

The government has published a Housing Green Paper *Quality and Choice: A Decent Home for All* (DETR 2000a). It has been criticized for being too timorous but it does present policies on rent harmonization, brings choice into allocation policies and addresses the huge repair backlog in the public and private sectors. These are all factors which promote the social inclusion of older people.

Making a reality of the preventive agenda

Increased targeting over the years of the new, post-1993, community care regime has, in theory, been reversed but the sums of money involved have been small and housing is usually involved only in the technical, narrow sense described by Allen (1997) in his critique of its role. However, the massive investment in the health service announced in the summer of 2000 must be welcomed (DoH 2000). The NHS is now expected to grow by one-half in cash terms and by one-third in real terms in just five years. These decisions firmly situate health in the community and hence strengthen the preventive role of the NHS.

All our recommendations for policy change hang together. If more was invested into housing and into urban regeneration as described above under *integrated social policy*, substantial savings could be made in health and social care budgets. The old adage 'prevention is better than cure' needs to adopt more of a housing spin. Moreover, housing has also a key role to play much later in the life course. We propose that anti-collective living attitudes are dispensed with in favour of an expansion of living situations chosen by older people, designed by older people and controlled by older people. There are situations where some older people will benefit and have healthier lives living together in a range of different living forms. These must not be seen as special needs housing. The current traditional forms of sheltered housing and residential care are full of defects. This recommendation about widening the opportunities for older people to live together when they choose to do so in various forms of supported housing by no means undermines the previous plea for more balanced communities which mix up age, tenure and so on. Indeed, it complements it. Within a balanced community there should be room for older people to live together. Age-segregated settings have been pilloried by the not old as discriminatory. They need not be. It is so unhelpful for community care to be crudely contrasted with residential care. The former means living in an existing home and is 'good'. The latter is bad. The contrast is too sharp. Older people with substantial resources for some time have opted to live together in some form or other of group living although, even for this group, the opportunities are limited. The opportunities for those without money are few; they are at the mercy of the ghost of the Charity Organization Society; assessed for and allocated to that form of living arrangement which is considered to be the cheaper in situations when someone else has decided it is no longer economic to care for the person in their own home. Chapter 7 showed that the newer forms of provision which are neither truly residential care nor truly sheltered housing can play an important preventive role. The concept of independent living seems to be much easier to deliver in housing rather than care-based forms of provision. In housing models the fundamental principle is that people have their 'own front door'.

Dealing with boundary issues

A consistent trend in the development of community care policies has been the attempt to separate care from accommodation. For examples the reforms of April 1993 were about taking the payment of residential care from the social security system and dividing it up into separate 'bits', accommodation, care and living costs. The *Supporting People* changes are about reducing housing benefit costs by disentangling housing from support. With this concept of separating accommodation from care we are back again with the idea that governments are good at deception. We, and many others, most certainly applaud the public rationale for these changes, that is, services should go to people. People should not have to move to get the services they want. Similarly we would support the notion that older people should be given more opportunities to choose and control. The separation of accommodation and care is justified in these terms. However, here is the power to deceive. In reality the separation is far less about user empowerment and much more about imposing boundaries to control individual government departments' costs. The evidence we have considered makes us believe that the government was wrong to reject the key proposal of the Royal Commission that both health and social care should be free at the point of consumption and paid through general taxation (DoH 2000). As it is, every person who has to consider residential care must continue to seek advice about how to avoid the worst financial penalties, and hours of professional advocacy will go into supporting each and every individual case.

Redefining joint working

For the messages of our book to be heeded, joint working has got to be reinvented. It has to work better than it has in the past. However, joint working is probably the most intractable problem raised in this book. All exhortations in the past have largely failed. The present Labour government has paid a great deal of attention to joint working and there are some successes, but the future does not look necessarily good for the continued involvement of housing. The NHS Plan (DoH 2000) places health at the centre of and in charge of community care. This could marginalize housing. Furthermore, in the plan the government rejects the Royal Commission's recommendation that personal care should be funded out of general taxation. We see no logical reason for the separation of health and social care. Once again it can make joint working harder. We also deplore the fact that health care is 'free' and social care is not.

Our final comment is that joint working will improve only if all agencies at all levels embrace the idea of genuine independent living, embrace the notion of empowerment and abandon the medical model. If this could happen the aspirations and preferences of older people themselves would not be out of kilter with those of professionals.

Redefining housing need

The most important message of this book is that the concept of older people's housing need should be completely redrawn so that it embraces the following:

- the majority, not just those living in specialized housing
- people living in rural areas, which means including the issue of transport
- those often neglected, including black and ethnic minority older people and tenants in the private rented sector, who outnumber the tenants of housing associations
- the concept that housing intervention long before later life performs a preventive function
- equity between tenures, a very obvious example being in the delivery of adaptations where people living in rented housing may receive less favourable treatment than owner-occupiers, or moving, where owners may be barred from local authority help
- a focus on the importance of space rather than a concentration only on issues to do with access
- allocation policies which operate a wide definition of housing need, for example, recognizing the importance of neighbourhoods to older people
- the need for accessible, barrier-free housing and more resources in the mean time for adaptations
- an appreciation of the fact that living successfully at home requires a wide notion of housing service to include cleaning, decorating, housework, gardening, companionship and shopping. These low-level preventive services do not necessarily have to be delivered by housing providers but they are salient to maintaining life in ordinary housing. Their delivery requires effective joint working.

Concluding comment

As this book ends, we ask the reader to stand back and consider again for themselves the great array of citizens aged from 55 to 105 (or more) living in every form of housing from inner city high-rise block to isolated highland farm, serving society in a rich variety of ways, as workers paid and unpaid, as neighbours and employers, as gardeners and creative artists, and as parents, grandparents and other guardians of the coming generations. When such a panorama is considered, it will be evident that society's provision of housing and housing services for older people must break away from the provision of 'cupboards' and 'care' for a deserving few and become mainstream, broadranging, creative and forward looking.

What we are proposing is a social model of later life to replace the present medical model. We suggest a move away from cash-limited budgets to a more rights-based system in the belief that this will not open Pandora's box.

We believe there should be less reliance on assessment and more emphasis on trusting older people's ability to say what they want, and for those with more complex needs we call for assessment or approaches which are holistic and which are centred upon the aspirations of older people. The available evidence is that this leads to a more cost-effective use of resources. Above all we require the definition of housing need to be broadened out to include the provision of low-level, preventive services. Finally, effective joint working is crucial to our grand plan if a seamless service is to be achieved.

References

Acheson, Sir Donald (1998) *Independent Inquiry into Inequalities*, Acheson Report. London: DoH.

Age Concern (1998) *Beyond Bricks and Mortar: Dignity and Security in the Home: Submission to the Royal Commission Long Term Care*. London: Age Concern.

Age Concern England and RADAR (1999) *Disabled Facilities Grants: Is the System Working?* A survey by Age Concern and RADAR. London: Age Concern England and RADAR.

Age Concern Scotland, Angus Council Housing and Social Work, Perth and Kinross Housing and Social Work, Scottish Homes, Tayside Health (1997) *Provision of Housing and Care Services for Older People in Rural Angus and Perth and Kinross: Report of Research Findings* Edinburgh: Published by the commissioning bodies as listed.

Allen, C. (1997) The policy and implementation of the housing role in community care: a constructionist theoretical perspective, *Housing Studies*, 12(1): 85–110.

Allen, C., Clapham, D., Franklin, B. and Parker, J. (1998) *The Right Home? Assessing Housing Needs in Community Care*. Cardiff: Centre of Housing Management and Development, Department of City and Regional Planning, Cardiff University.

Allen, I., Hogg, D. and Peace, S. (1992) *Elderly People: Choice, Participation and Satisfaction*. London: Policy Studies Institute.

Anchor Trust (1998) *Killer Homes: Facing Up to Poor Housing as a Cause of Older People's Ill-Health*. Oxford: Anchor Trust.

Arblaster, L., Conway, J., Foreman, A. and Hawtin, M. (1996) *Asking the Impossible? Inter-Agency Working to Address Housing, Health and Social Care Needs of People in Ordinary Housing*. Bristol: Policy Press.

Askham, J., Nelson, H., Tinker, A. and Hancock, R. (1999) *To Have and to Hold: The Bond Between Older People and the Homes They Own*. York: York Publishing Services.

Audit Commission (1996) *Balancing the Care Equation*. London: Audit Commission.

Audit Commission (1997) *The Coming of Age: Improving Care Services for Older People*. Abingdon: Audit Commission.

Audit Commission (1998) *Home Alone: The Role of Housing in Community Care*. London: Audit Commission.

Avila, D.L. and Combs, A.W. (eds) (1985) *Perspectives on Helping Relationships and the Helping Professions, Past Present and Future.* Boston, MA: Allyn and Bacon.

Baldwin, N., Harris, J. and Kelly, D. (1993) Institutionalisation: why blame the institution? *Ageing and Society*, 13(1): 69–81.

Barnes, C., Mercer, G. and Shakespeare, T. (1999) *Exploring Disability: A Sociological Introduction.* Oxford: Polity.

Barnes, M. and Bennett-Emslie, G. (1997) *If They Would Listen: An Evaluation of the Fife User Panels.* Edinburgh: Age Concern Scotland.

Beck, U. (1992) *The Risk Society.* London: Sage.

Benjamin, D. and Stea, D. (eds) (1995) *The Home: Words, Interpretations, Meanings and Environments.* Aldershot: Avebury.

Bernard, M. and Phillips, J. (2000) The challenge of ageing in tomorrow's Britain, *Ageing and Society*, 20(1): 33–54.

Better Government for Older People Steering Committee (2000) *All Our Futures.* Wolverhampton: Better Government for Older People Programme.

Biggs, S., Philipson, C. and Kingston, P. (1993) *Old Age Abuse.* Buckingham: Open University Press.

Blakemore, K. (2000) Health and social care in minority communities: an over problematized issue?, *Health and Social Care in the Community*, 8(1): 22–30.

Blakemore, K. and Boneham, M. (1994) *Age, Race and Ethnicity: A Comparative Approach.* Buckingham: Open University Press.

Bond, J., Coleman, P. and Peace, S. (1993) *Ageing in Society: An Introduction to Social Gerontology*, 2nd edn. London: Sage.

Booth, C. (1894) *The Aged Poor in England and Wales: Condition.* London: Macmillan.

Booth, T. (1985) *Home Truths: Old People's Homes and the Outcome of Care.* Aldershot: Gower.

Brenton, M. (1998) *Co Housing Communities of Older People in the Netherlands: Lessons for Britain?* Bristol: Policy Press.

Burholt, V. (1997) Testing behavioural and developmental models of migration: a re-evaluation of migration patterns among the elderly and why older people move, *Environment and Planning* A, 31: 2071–88.

Burnett, J. (1986) *A Social History of Housing*, 2nd edn. London: Methuen.

Burridge, R. and Ormandy, D. (eds) (1993) *Unhealthy Housing: Research, Remedies and Reforms.* London: Spon.

Burrows, R. (1999) The contemporary dynamics of residualisation: an analysis of residential mobility, social exclusion and social housing in England, *Journal of Social Policy*, 28(1): 27–52.

Butler, A., Oldman, C. and Greve, J. (1983) *Sheltered Housing for the Elderly: Policy, Practice and the Consumer.* London: Allen & Unwin.

Bytheway, B. (1995) *Ageism.* Buckingham: Open University Press.

Campbell, J. and Oliver, M. (1996) *Disability Politics: Understanding our Past, Changing our Future.* London: Routledge.

Care and Repair England (1999) Home improvement agency managing organisations, *Care and Repair England Newsletter*, 64, Nov/Dec.

Carter, T. and Nash, C. (1995) Pensioning forums – a voice for older people, in R. Jack (ed.) *Empowerment in Community Care.* London: Chapman and Hall.

Cebulla, A., with Beach, J., Heaver, C., Irving, Z., Walker, R. and the National Centre for Social Research (1999) *Housing Benefit and Supported Accommodation*, Department of Social Security Research Report no. 93. Leeds: Corporate Document Services.

Challis, D. and Bartlett, H. (1987) *Old and Ill: Private Nursing Homes for Elderly People.* London: Age Concern Institute of Gerontology.

Chapman, T. and Hockey, J. (eds) (1999) *Ideal Homes? Social Change and Domestic Life.* London: Routledge.

Clapham, D. (1997) Problems and potential of sheltered housing, *Ageing and Society,* 17(2): 209–14.

Clapham, D. and Franklin, B. (1994) *The Housing Management Contribution to Community Care.* University of Glasgow: Centre for Housing Research and Urban Studies.

Clapham, D. and Munro, M. (1988) *A Comparison of Sheltered and Amenity Housing for Older People.* Edinburgh: Scottish Office.

Clapham, D. and Munro, M. (1990) Ambiguities and contradiction in the provision of sheltered housing for older people, *Journal of Social Policy,* 19(1): 27–45.

Clapham, D. and Smith, S. (1990) Housing policy and special needs, *Policy and Politics,* 18(3): 193–206.

Clapham, D., Means, R. and Munro, M. (1993) Housing, the life course and older people, in S. Arber and M. Evandrou (eds) *Ageing, Independence and the Life Course.* London: Jessica Kingsley.

Clapham, D., Munro, M. and Kay, H. (1994) *A Wider Choice: Revenue Funding Mechanisms, Housing and Community Care.* York: Joseph Rowntree Foundation.

Clark, H., Dyer, S. and Hartman, L. (1996) *Going Home: Older People Leaving Hospital.* Bristol: Policy Press.

Clark, H., Dyer, S. and Horwood, J. (1998) *That Bit of Help.* Bristol: Policy Press.

Clough, R. (1997) *Living in Someone Else's Home: The Concept of Negotiation, the Process of Ownership and the Role of Relationships in Homes for Older People.* London: Counsel and Care.

Coleman, P. (1994) Adjustments in later life, in J. Bond, P. Coleman and S. Peace (eds) *Ageing in Society.* London: Sage.

Coles, A. (1989) How often do people move house?, *Housing Finance,* 4: 15.

Cooper, L., Watson, L. and Allen, G. (1994) *Shared Living: Social Relations in Supported Housing.* Social Services Monographs, Research in Practice. Sheffield: Joint Unit for Social Services Research and Community Care, University of Sheffield.

Cowan, D. and Turner-Smith, A. (1999) The role of assistance technology in alternative models of care for older people. Appendix 4 of *Alternative Models of Care for Older People.* Research Volume 2 of the Royal Commission Report with Respect to Hold Age. London: Stationery Office.

Crane, M. (1999) *Understanding Older Homeless People.* Buckingham: Open University Press.

Crotch, W. (1908) *The Cottage Homes of England: The Case Against the Housing System in Rural Districts,* 3rd edn. London: Industrial Publishing Company.

Cumming, E. and Henry, W. (1961) *Growing Old: The Process of Disengagement.* New York: Basic Books.

D'Aboville, E. (1994) *Promoting User Involvement.* London: King's Fund.

Deakin, N. (1995) The perils of partnership: the voluntary sector and the state 1945–1992, in J. Davis Smith, C. Rochester and R. Hedley (eds) *An Introduction to the Voluntary Sector,* London: Routledge.

Department of the Environment (DoE) (1993) *English House Condition Survey 1991,* London: HMSO.

Department of the Environment (DoE) (1995) *Housing Strategies: Guidance for Local Authorities on the Preparation of Housing Strategies.* London: HMSO.

Department of the Environment (DoE) (1997) *Housing Grants, Construction and Regeneration Act.* London: Stationery Office.

Department of the Environment and Department of Health (DoE/DoH) (1990) *House Adaptations for People with Disabilities,* Joint Circular 10/90 (DoE) LAC(90)7 (DoH). London: HMSO.

Department of the Environment and Department of Health (DoE/DoH) (1996) *Code of Guidance in Parts VI and VII of the Housing Act 1996*. London: HMSO.

Department of the Environment, Transport and the Regions (DETR) (1998a) *Modernising Local Government: Improving Local Services through Best Value*. London: Stationery Office.

Department of the Environment, Transport and the Regions (DETR) (1998b) Housing fitness standard: a consultation paper (www.housing.detr.gov.uk/consult/hfs/) (updated 17 February 1998).

Department of the Environment, Transport and the Regions (DETR) (1998c) Circular 8/98 (WO 32/98): The Building Act 1984 – The Building Regulations (Amendment) Regulations 1998: new part M in Schedule 1 to the Building Regulations 1991. London: Stationery Office.

Department of the Environment, Transport and the Regions (DETR) (1999a) *Tenant Participation Compacts: Consultation Paper*. London: Stationery Office.

Department of the Environment, Transport and the Regions (DETR) (1999b) *Housing and Construction Statistics 1988–98*. London: Government Statistical Service.

Department of the Environment, Transport and the Regions (DETR) (2000a) *Quality and Choice: A Decent Home for All*. London: DETR.

Department of the Environment, Transport and the Regions (DETR) (2000b) *Housing and Construction Statistics*: March quarter. London: Stationery Office.

Department of Health (DoH) (1970) *Chronically Sick and Disabled People's Act*. London: DoH.

Department of Health (DoH) (1989) *Caring for People: Community Care in the Next Decade and Beyond*, Cm 849. London: HMSO.

Department of Health (DoH) (1990) *Caring for People: Community Care in the Next Decade and Beyond Policy Guidance*. London: HMSO.

Department of Health (DoH) (1994a) *The F Factor: Reasons Why Some Older People Choose Residential Care*. London: DoH.

Department of Health (DoH) (1994b) *Hospital Discharge Workbook: A Manual on Hospital Discharge Practice*. London: DoH.

Department of Health (DoH) (1995) *Building Bridges: A Guide to Arrangements for Inter-Agency Working for the Care and Protection of Severely Mentally Ill People*. London: HMSO.

Department of Health (DoH) (1997a) *The New NHS: Modern and Dependable*. London: Stationery Office.

Department of Health (DoH) (1997b) *Better Services for Vulnerable People*. London: DoH.

Department of Health (DoH) (1998a) *Modernising Social Services: Promoting Independence, Improving Production, Raising Standards*. London: Stationery Office.

Department of Health (DoH) (1998b) *Our Healthier Nation: A Contract for Health*. London: Stationery Office.

Department of Health (DoH) (1998c) *Partnership in Action: New Opportunities for Joint Working between Health and Social Services A Discussion Document*. London: DoH.

Department of Health (DoH) (1998d) *Modernising Health and Social Services: National Priorities Guidance 1999/000 2001/02*. London: DoH.

Department of Health (DoH) (1998e) *Better Services for Vulnerable People Maintaining the Momentum*, (to be completed).

Department of Health (DoH) (1999a) *Saving Lives: Our Healthier Nation*. London: Stationery Office.

Department of Health (DoH) (1999b) *Housing and Community Care: Establishing a Strategic Framework*. London: DoH.

Department of Health (DoH) (2000) *The NHS Plan: A Plan for Investment, a Plan for Reform*. London: Stationery Office.

Department of Health and Department of the Environment (DoH/DoE) (1997) *Housing and Community Care: Establishing a Strategic Framework*. London: DoH.

Department of Health and Department of the Environment, Transport and the Regions (DoH/DETR) (1999) Health Act 1999 – Modern Partnerships for the People. Letter to key health and social care agencies, 8 September. London: DoH/DETR.

Department of Social Security (DSS) (1998a) *A New Contract for Pensions: Partnerships in Pensions*. London: Stationery Office.

Department of Social Security (DSS) (1998b) *Supporting People: A Policy and Funding Framework for Support Services*. London: DSS.

Dominelli, L. and Hoogvelt, A. (1996) Globalization and the technocratisition of social work, *Critical Social Policy*, 16(2): 45–62.

Druce, N. (2000) Improving assessment of core needs for older people, local authority perspective: rapid response system. Paper given at Laing and Buisson conference, Improving Assessment of Care Needs of Older People, London, 24 May.

Dupuis, A. and Thorns, D. (1996) Meaning home has for older people, *Housing Studies*, 11(4): 485–501.

England, J., Oldman, C. and Hearnshaw, S. (2000) *A Question of Shared Care? The Role of Relatives in Sheltered Housing*. Oxford: Anchor Trust.

Ernst and Young (1994) *The Cost of Specialised Housing*, Housing Research Report no. 2. London: DoE.

Estes, C. (1979) *The Ageing Enterprise*. San Francisco, CA: Jossey Bass.

Estes, C. (1986) The politics of ageing in America, *Ageing and Society*, 6(2): 121–34.

Evandrou, M. (ed.) (1997) *Baby Boomers: Ageing in the 21st Century*. London: Age Concern.

Falkingham, J. (1997) Who are the baby boomers? A demographic profile, in M. Evandrou (ed.) *Baby Boomers: Ageing in the 21st Century*. London: Age Concern.

Featherstone, M. and Hepworth, M. (1989) Ageing and old age: reflections on the postmodern life course, in B. Bytheway, T. Keil, P. Allat and A. Bryman (eds) *Becoming and Being Old*. London: Sage.

Fletcher, P. (2000) *Social Inclusion for Vulnerable People: Linking Regeneration and Community Care – The Housing, Care and Support Dimension*. Brighton: Pavilion.

Fletcher, P., Riseborough, M., Humphries, J., Jenkins, C. and Whittingham, P. (1999) *Citizenship and Services in Old Age: The Strategic Role of Very Sheltered Housing*. Beaconsfield: Housing 21.

Flynn, N. (1989) The 'new right' and social policy, *Policy and Politics*, 17(2): 97–110.

Foucault, M. (1967) *Madness and Civilisation*. London: Routledge.

Foucault, M. (1977) *Discipline and Punish*. London: Allen Lane.

Giddens, A. (1979) *Critical Problems in Social Theory*. London: Macmillan.

Giddens, A. (1991) *Modernity and Self Identity*. Cambridge: Polity.

Gilleard, C. (1996) Consumption and identity in later life: toward a cultural gerontology, *Ageing and Society*, 16(4): 489–98.

Ginn, J. and Arber, S. (1996) Gender, age and attitudes to retirement in mid life, *Ageing and Society*, 16(1): 27–55.

Glendinning, C. and Wilkin, D. (1999) Primary health care in health and welfare systems, *Health and Social Care: The Community*, 7(5): 311–15.

Goffman, E. (1961) *Asylums*. Hardmondsworth: Penguin.

Goldsmith, M. (1996) *Hearing the Voice of People with Dementia: Opportunities and Obstacles*. London: Jessica Kingsley.

Greenwood, C. and Smith, J. (1999) *Sharing in Extra Care*. Staines: Hanover Housing Group.

Griffiths, R. (1988) *Community Care: An Agenda for Action*. London: HMSO.

Griffiths, S. (1997) *Housing Benefit and Supported Housing: The Implications of Recent Changes*. York: Joseph Rowntree Foundation.

Gubrium, J. (1986) *Oldtimers and Alzheimer's: The Descriptive Organisation of Senility*. Greenwich, CT: JAI Press.

Gubrium, J. (1993) *Speaking of Life: Horizons of Meaning for Nursing Home Residents*. New York: Aldine de Gruyter.

Gurney, C. and Means, P. (1993) The meaning of home in later life, in S. Arthur and M. Evandrou (eds) *Ageing, Independence and the Life Crises*. London: Jessica Kingsley.

Hadley, R. and Clough, R. (1996) *Care in Chaos: Frustration and Challenge in Community Care*. London: Cassell.

Hancock, R. (1997) Financial resources in later life, in M. Evandrou (ed.) *Baby Boomers: Ageing in the 21st Century*. London: Age Concern.

Hancock, R. (2000) Estimating the housing wealth of older home owners in Britain, *Housing Studies*, 15(4): 561–80.

Harding, T. (1997) *A Life Worth Living*. London: Help the Aged.

Harrison, L. and Heywood, F. (2000) *Health Begins at Home: Planning at the Health – Housing Interface for Older People*. Bristol: Policy Press.

Harrison, L. and Means, R. (1990) *Housing: The Essential Element in Community Care*. Oxford: Anchor Housing Trust.

Hasler, J. and Page, D. (1998) *Sheltered Housing is Changing: The Emerging Role of the Warden*. Nottingham: Metropolitan Housing Trust.

Hasler, F., Campbell, J. and Zarb, G. (2000) *Direct Routes to Independence: A Guide to Local Authority Implementation of Direct Payments*. London: Policy Studies Institute.

Havinghurst, M. (1954) Flexibility and the social roles of the retired, *American Journal of Sociology*, 59(1/2): 309–11.

Hawes, D. (1997) *Older People and Homelessness*. Bristol: Policy Press.

Health and Housing (1998) *Towards a Strategy for Health and Housing*. London: Health and Housing.

Help the Aged (1992) *Growing Old in the Countryside*. London: Help the Aged.

Heywood, F. (1993) *Housing Option Appraisal Method (Hoamchoice)*. Bristol: School of Advanced Urban Studies for Community Forum, Birmingham.

Heywood, F. (1997) Poverty and disrepair, *Housing Studies*, 12(1): 27–46.

Heywood, F. (2001) *Money Well Spent: The Effectiveness and Value of Housing Adaptations*. Bristol: Policy Press.

Heywood, F. and Naz, M. (1990) *Clearance: The View from the Street*. Birmingham: Community Forum.

Heywood, F. and Smart, G. (1996) *Funding Adaptations*. Bristol: Policy Press.

Heywood, F., Pate, A., Means, R. and Galvin, J. (1999) *Housing Options for Older People (Hoop): Report on a Developmental Project to Refine a Housing Option Appraisal Tool for Use by Older People*. London: Elderly Accommodation Counsel.

Higgins, J. (1989) Defining community care: realities and myths, *Social Policy and Administration*, 23(2): 3–16.

Higgs, P. (1995) Citizenship and old age: the end of the road, *Ageing and Society*, 15(4): 535–50.

Hill, O. (1998) *Octavia Hill and the Social Housing Debate: Essays and Letters by Octavia Hill*, edited by Robert Whelan. London: Health and Welfare Unit, Institute of Economic Affairs.

Hills, J. (1993) *The Future of Welfare: A Guide to the Debate*. York: Joseph Rowntree Foundation.

HOPe (Health and Older People Group) (2000) *Our Future Health: Older People's Priorities for Health and Social Care*. London: Help the Aged.

Hornby, S. (1993) *Collaborative Care: Interprofessional, Interagency and Interpersonal.* Oxford: Blackwell.

Hudson, B. (1987) Collaboration in social welfare: a framework for analysis, *Policy and Politics*, 15(3): 174–82.

Hudson, B. (1999) Primary health care and social care working, *Managing Community Care*, 7(1): 15–22.

Hughes, D. and Wilkin, D. (1987) Physical care and the quality of life in residential care, *Ageing and Society*, 7(4): 399–426.

Hughes, S. (2000) The surgery, *Housing*, Dec/Jan: 11.

Hunt, A. (1970) *The Home-Help Service in England and Wales.* London: HMSO.

Huxham, C. (ed.) (1996) *Creating Collaborative Advantage.* London: Sage.

Jamieson, A., Harper, S. and Victor, C. (1997) *Critical Approaches to Ageing and Later Life.* Buckingham: Open University Press.

Jacobs, T. (1978) *Older Persons and Retirement Communities.* Springfield, Il: Thomas.

Jerrome, D. (1992) *Good Company: An Anthropological Study of Old People in Groups.* Edinburgh: Edinburgh University Press.

Johnson, M. (1976) That was your life: a biographical approach to later life, in J. Munnichs and W. Van Den Heuval (eds) *Dependency and Interdependency in Old Age.* The Hague: Martinus Nijhoff.

Jones, N. (1999) *I Never Thought I'd Be Doing This: Older People Networking – An Evaluation of Anchor Trust's Local Service Network Projects.* Oxford: Anchor Trust.

Jorm, A. and Korten, A. (1988) A method for calculating projected increases in the number of dementia sufferers, *Australian and New Zealand Journal of Psychiatry*, 22(2): 183–9.

Karn, V. (1977) *Retiring to the Seaside.* London: Routledge and Kegan Paul.

Kitwood, T. and Benson, S. (1995) *The New Culture of Dementia Care.* London: Hawker.

Kitwood, T., Buckland, S. and Petrie, T. (1995) *Brighter Futures.* Oxford: Anchor Trust.

Laing and Buisson (1997) *Housing with Care in the UK: From Sheltered Housing to Assisted Living.* London: Laing and Buisson.

Laing and Buisson (1998) *Care of Elderly People: Market Survey*, 11th edn. London: Laing and Buisson.

Langan, J. and Means, R. (1995) *Personal Finances Elderly People with Dementia and the 'New' Community Care.* Oxford: Anchor Trust.

Langan, J., Means, R. and Rolfe, S. (1996) *Maintaining Home and Independence in Later Life: Older People Speaking.* Oxford: Anchor Trust.

Leather, P. (1993) *Renovation File.* Oxford: Anchor Trust.

Leather, P. (1999) *Age File '99.* Oxford: Anchor Trust.

Leather, P. and Mackintosh, S. (1992) *Maintaining Home Ownership: The Agency Approach.* London: Longman.

Leonard, P. (1982) Introduction, in C. Phillipson, *Capitalism and the Construction of Old Age.* London: Macmillan.

Lewis, H., Fletcher, P., Hardy, B., Milne, A. and Waddington, E. (1999) *Promoting Wellbeing: Developing a Preventive Approach with Older People.* Oxford: Anchor Trust.

Litwak, E. and Longino, C.F. (1987) Migration patterns among the elderly: a developmental perspective, *The Gerontologist*, 27(3): 266–72.

Lloyd, L. (2000) Dying in old age: promoting well being at the end of life, *Mortality*, 5(2): 176–88.

Loch, C.S. (1911) Charity and charities, in *Encyclopedia Britannica*, vol. V, pp. 884–91. Cambridge: Cambridge University Press.

Lord Chancellor's Department (1997) *Who Decides? Making Decisions on Behalf of Mentality Incapacitated Adults*, Cm 3803. London: Lord Chancellor's Department.

Lowe, R. (1999) *The Welfare State in Britain since 1945.* London: Macmillan.

Lynott, R. and Lynott, P. (1996) Tracing the course of theoretical development in the sociology of ageing, *The Gerontologist*, 36(6): 749–60.

McCafferty, P. (1994) *Living Independently: A Study of the Housing Needs of Elderly and Disabled People.* London: HMSO.

McKenzie, E. (1994) *Privatopia: Homeowner Associations and the Rise of Residential Private Government.* New Haven, CT and London: Yale University Press.

Mackintosh, S. and Leather, P. (1992) *Staying Put Revisited.* Oxford: Anchor Housing Trust.

Mackintosh, S., Means, R. and Leather, P. (1990) *Housing in Later Life: The Housing Finance Implications of an Ageing Society.* Bristol: School of Advanced Urban Studies.

Malpass, P. and Murie, A. (1999) *Housing Policy and Practice*, 5th edn. London: Macmillan.

Marsh, A. and Riseborough, M. (1995) *Making Ends Meet: Older People, Housing Costs and the Affordability of Rented Housing.* London: National Federation of Housing Association.

Marsh, A., Gordon, D., Heslop, P. and Pantazis, C. (2000) Housing deprivation and health: a longitudinal analysis, *Housing Studies*, 15(3): 411–28.

Marshall, T.H. (1992) *Citizenship and Social Class.* London: Pluto.

Means, R. (1987) Older people in British housing studies: rediscovery and emerging issues for research, *Housing Studies*, 2(2): 82–98.

Means, R. (1996) Housing and community care for older people: joint working at the local level, *Journal of Inter-professional Care*, 10(3): 273–83.

Means, R. (1997a) Home, independence and community care: time for a wider vision?, *Policy and Politics*, 25(4): 409–20.

Means, R. (1997b) Housing options in 2020 a suitable home for all?, in M. Evandrou (ed.) *Baby Boomers: Ageing in the 21st Century.* London: Age Concern.

Means, R. (1999) Housing and housing organisations: a review of their contribution to alternative models of care for elderly people. Appendix 3 of *Alternative Models of Care for Older People*, Research Volume 2 of the Royal Commission Report. London: Stationery Office.

Means, R. and Smith, R. (1998a) *Community Care: Policy and Practice*, 2nd edn. London: Macmillan.

Means, R. and Smith, R. (1998b) *From Poor Law to Community Care: The Development of Welfare Services for Elderly People, 1939–71.* Bristol: Policy Press.

Means, R., Brenton, M., Harrison, L. and Heywood, F. (1997) *Making Partnerships Work in Community Care: A Guide for Practitioners in Housing, Health and Social Services.* Bristol: Policy Press.

Mellett, A. (1996) *Room to Manouevre: A Study of Under Occupation, With Particular Reference to North Devon.* MA dissertation, University of the West of England.

Merrett, S. (1979) *State Housing in Britain.* London: Routledge and Kegan Paul.

Middleton, L. (1981) *So Much for So Few: A View of Sheltered Housing.* Liverpool: Institute of Human Ageing, University of Liverpool.

Midgeley, G., Munlo, I. and Brown, M. (1997) *Sharing Power: Integrating User Involvement and Multi-Agency Working to Improve Housing for Older People.* Bristol: Policy Press.

Midwinter, E. (1992) *Citizenship: From Ageism to Participation.* The Carnegie Inquiry into the Third Age, Research Paper no. 8, Dunfermline.

Milne, A. (1999) *Later Lifestyles: A Survey by Help the Aged Yours Magazine.* London: Help the Aged.

Minkler, M. (1996) Critical perspectives on ageing: new challenges for gerontology, *Ageing and Society*, 16(4): 467–87.

Moody, H. (1988) Towards a critical gerontology: the contribution of the humanities to theories of ageing, in J. Birren and V. Bengston (eds) *Emergent Theories of Ageing*. New York: Springer.

Moroney, R. (1976) *The Family and the State*. London: Longman.

Morris, J. (1991) *Pride against Prejudice: Transforming Attitudes to Disability*. London: Women's Press.

National Federation of Housing Associations (NFHA) (1994) *Housing Associations in the Community Care Market Place*. London: NFHA.

Neill, J., Sinclair, I., Gorbach, P. and Williams, J. (1988) *A Need for Care: Elderly Applicants for Local Authority Homes*. Aldershot: Gower.

Netten, A. and Dennett, J. (1997) *Unit Costs of Health and Social Care*. Canterbury: Personal Social Services Unit, University of Kent.

Netten, A., Bibbington, A., Darton, R., Forder, J. and Miles, K. (1998) *Survey of Care Homes for Elderly People*. Canterbury: Personal Social Services, University of Kent.

Nettleton, S. and Watson, J. (eds) (1998) *The Body in Everyday Life*. London: Routledge.

Neugarten, B. and Hagestad, G. (1976) Age and the life course, in R. Burstock and E. Shonas (eds) *Handbook of Ageing and the Social Sciences*. New York: Van Nostrand Reinhold.

Nocon, A. (1989) Forms of ignorance and their role in the joint planning process, *Social Policy and Administration*, 23(1): 31–47

Nocon, A. and Pleace, N. (1999) Sheltered housing and community care, *Social Policy and Administration*, 23(2): 164–80.

Nocon, A. and Qureshi, H. (1996) *Outcomes of Community Care for Users and Carers: Social Services Perspectives*. Buckingham: Open University Press.

Oberg, P. (1996) The absent body: a social gerontological paradox, *Ageing and Society*, 16(6): 701–19.

Office for National Statistics (ONS) (1996) *Housing in England 1994/95*. London: HMSO.

Office for National Statistics (1997) *Housing in England 1995/96*. London: Stationery Office.

Office for National Statistics (ONS) (1999a) *Family Spending*. London: Stationery Office.

Office for National Statistics (ONS) (1999b) *General Household Survey 1996*. London: Stationery Office.

Office for National Statistics (ONS) (1999c) *Annual Abstract of Statistics* no. 135, 1999 edn. London: Stationery Office.

Office of Population Census and Surveys and General Register; Office Scotland (OPCS) (1994) *1991 Census: Key Statistics for Local Authorities*. London: HMSO.

Office of Population Census and Surveys and General Register; Office Scotland (OPCS) (1995) *The 1991 Census of Great Britain: General Report*. London: HMSO.

O'Hagan, G. (1999) *Of Primary Importance: Inspection of Social Services Departments' Links with Primary Health Services Older People*. London: DH (Social Services Inspectorate).

Oldman, C. (1988) More than bricks and mortar, *Housing*, 24(5): 13–16.

Oldman, C. (1990) *Moving in Old Age: New Directions in Housing Policies*. London: HMSO.

Oldman, C. (1991a) *Paying for Care: Personal Sources of Funding Care*. York: Joseph Rowntree Foundation.

Oldman, C. (1991b) Financial effects of moving in old age, *Housing Studies*, 6(4): 251–62.

Oldman, C. (2000a) *Developing a Housing and Community Care Strategy for Older People: A Do it Yourself Guide*. Oxford: Anchor Trust.

Oldman, C. (2000b) *Blurring the Boundaries: A Fresh Look at Housing Provision and Care for Older People*. Brighton: Pavilion.

Oldman, C. and Beresford, B. (2000) Home, sick home: using the housing experience of disabled children to suggest a new theoretical framework, *Housing Studies*, 15(3): 429–42.

Oldman, C. and Quilgars, D. (1999) The last resort? Revisiting ideas about older people's living arrangements, *Ageing and Society*, 19(4): 363–84.

Oliver, M. (1990) *The Politics of Disablement*. London: Macmillan.

Oliver, M. (1992) Changing the social relations of research production, *Disability, Handicap and Society*, 7(2): 101–11

Oliver, M. (1996) *Understanding Disability: From Theory to Practice*. London: Macmillan.

Owens, P., Carrier, J. and Horder, J. (eds) (1995) *Inter-professional Issues in Community and Primary Health Care*. London: Macmillan.

Parker, G. (1993) *With this Body: Caring and Disability in Marriage*. Buckingham: Open University Press.

Patel, N. (1999) Black and Minority Ethnic Elders: Perspectives on Long Term Care. Research Volume 1 of the *Royal Commission Report With Respect to Old Age: Long Term Care: Rights and Responsibilities*. London: Stationery Office.

Peace, S. (1993) The living environments of older women, in M. Bernard and K. Meade (eds) *Women Come of Age*. London: Edward Arnold.

Peace, S., Kellaher, L. and Willcocks, D. (1997) *Re-evaluating Residential Care*. Buckingham: Open University Press.

Phillips, T., Means, R., Russell, L. and Sykes, R. (eds) (1999) *Broadening our Vision of Community Care for Older People: Innovative Examples from Finland, Swindon and England*. Oxford: Anchor Trust.

Phillipson, C. (1998) *Reconstructing Old Age: New Agendas in Social Theory and Practice*. London: Sage.

Phillipson, C. and Walker, A. (eds) (1986) *Ageing and Social Policy: A Critical Assessment*. Aldershot: Gower.

Phillipson, C. and Walker, A. (1987) The case for critical gerontology, in S. Di Gergorio (ed.) *Social Gerontology: New Directions*. London: Croom Helm.

Plank, D. (1977) *Caring for the Elderly: Report of a Study of Caring for Dependent Elderly People in Eight London Boroughs*. London: Greater London Council.

Powell, M. (ed.) (1999) *New Labour, New Welfare State?* Bristol: Policy Press.

Pressman, J. and Wildavsky, A. (1973) *Implementation*. Berkeley, CA: University of California Press.

Reed, J. and Payton, V. (1996) Constructing familiarity and managing self: ways of adapting to life in nursing and residential homes for older people, *Ageing and Society*, 16(5): 543–60.

Rickford, F. (2000) The new IT generation, *Community Care*, 27 July–2 August: 18–19.

Riseborough, M. (1999) Representation and older citizens: their inclusion and exclusion. Paper presented to British Society of Gerontology Annual Conference, University of Bournemouth/University of Southampton 16th–18th September.

Riseborough, M. (2000) *Overlooked and Excluded: Older People and Regeneration*. London: Anchor Trust.

Rowntree, B. S. (1902) *Poverty: A Study of Town Life*, 4th edn. London: Macmillan (first published 1901).

Royal Commission (1999) *With Respect to Old Age: A Report by the Royal Commission on Long Term Care*. London: Stationery Office.

Royal Institute of Chartered Surveyors (RICS) (1997) *The Real Costs of Poor Housing*. Coventry: RICS.

Rudd, T. (1988) Basic problems in the social welfare of the elderly, *The Medical Officer*, 29 June: 348–9.

Rugg, J. (2000) *Hartrigg Oaks: The Early Development of a Continuing Care Community 1983–1999*. York: Centre for Housing Policy.

Rummery, K. and Glendinning, C. (1999) Negotiating needs, access and gatekeeping, *Critical Social Policy*, 19(3): 335–54.

Russell, L. (1999) *The Future of the Built Environment*. Debate of the Age Millennium Papers. London: Age Concern.

Ruth, J. and Kenyon, G. (1996) Introduction to special issue on ageing, biography and practice, *Ageing and Society*, 16(6): 653–8.

Sanders, W. (1903) *A Digest of the Results of the Census in England and Wales in 1901*. London: Charles and Edwin Layton.

Saunders, P. (1990) *A Nation of Home Owners*. London: Unwin and Hyman.

Seligman, M. (1975) *Helplessness*. New York: W.H. Freeman.

Shanas, E., Townsend, P., Wedderburn, D. *et al*. (1968) *Old People in Three Industrial Societies*. London: Routledge and Kegan Paul.

Shaw, V. (1999) *A Perfect Match? A Good Practice Guide to Disability Housing Registers*. London: Housing Corporation.

Sidell, M. (1995) *Health in Old Age: Myth, Mystery and Management*. Buckingham: Open University Press.

Simons, K. (1998) The regulation of housing and support services, *Housing, Care and Support*, 1(13): 10–15.

Sixsmith, A. (1990) The meaning and experience of 'home' in later life, in B. Bytheway and J. Johnson (eds) *Welfare and the Ageing Experience*. Aldershot: Avebury.

Smart, G. and Means, R. (1997) *Housing and Community Care: Exploring the Role of Home Improvement Agencies*. Oxford: Anchor Trust.

Smith, K. (1986) *I'm Not Complaining: The Housing Conditions of Elderly Private Tenants*. London: SHAC.

Smith, K. (1989) *Housing Agencies for Elderly Owner Occupiers*. London: SHAC.

Social Services Inspectorate (1994) *Occupational Therapy: The Community Contribution*. London: DH.

Steinfeld, E. (1981) The place of old age: the meaning of housing for old people, in J.S. Duncan (ed.).

Stewart, J., Harris, J. and Sapey, B. (1999) Disability and dependency: origins and failures of 'special needs' housing for disabled people, *Disability and Society*, 14(1): 5–20.

Swift, J. (1940) *Gulliver's Travels*. London: Dent.

Thane, P. (1998) The family lives of old people, in P. Johnson and P. Thane (eds) *Old Age from Antiquity to Postmodernity*. London: Routledge.

Thompson, D. and Page, D. (1999) *Effective Sheltered Housing: A Good Practice Guide*. London: Chartered Institute of Housing.

Tinker, A. (1989) *An Evaluation of Very Sheltered Housing*. London: HMSO.

Tinker, A., Wright, F. and Zeilig, H. (1995) *Difficult to Let Sheltered Housing*. London: HMSO.

Tinker, A., Wright, F., McCreadie, C. *et al*. (1999) Alternative models of care for older people, *Royal Commission on Long Term Care Research* vol. 2, Cm 4192–II/2. London: Stationery Office.

Toffaleti, C. for The Older People's Initiative (1997) *Voices for Choices: What Older People Say about their Housing – Examples of Good Practice in Housing and Linked Services*. Manchester: Greater Manchester, Centre for Voluntary Organisations.

Townsend, P. (1962) *The Last Refuge: A Survey of Residential Institutions and Homes for the Aged in England and Wales*. London: Routledge and Kegan Paul.

Townsend, P. (1963) *The Family Life of Old People*. Harmondsworth: Penguin.

Townsend, P. (1981) The structured dependency of the elderly: creation of social policy in the twentieth century, *Ageing and Society*, 1(1): 5–28.

Tozer, R. and Thornton, P. (1995) *A Meeting of Minds: Older People as Research Advisors*. York: Social Policy Research Unit, University of York.

Trotter, E. and Phillips, M. (1997) *Remodelling Sheltered Housing*. Beaconsfield: Housing 21.

Tulle-Winton, E. (1999) Growing old and resistance: towards a new cultural economy of old age? *Ageing and Society*, 19(3): 281–300.

Twigg, J. (1997) Deconstructing the 'social bath': help with bathing at home for old and disabled people, *Journal of Social Policy*, 26(2): 211–32.

Walker, A. (1981) Towards a political economy of old age, *Ageing and Society*, 1(1): 73–94.

Warnes, A.M. (1991) Migration to and seasonal residence in Spain of northern European elderly people, *European Journal of Gerontology and Geriatrics*, 1: 54–67.

Webb, A. (1991) Co-ordination, a problem in public sector management, *Policy and Politics*, 19(4): 29–42.

Wheeler, R. (1986) Housing policy and elderly people, in C. Phillipson and A. Walker (eds) *Ageing and Social Policy: A Critical Assessment*. Aldershot: Gower.

Wilcock, S. (1990) *Living with Alzheimer's Disease and Similar Conditions*. Harmondsworth: Penguin.

Wilcox, S. (1997) *Housing Finance Review 1997/98*. York: Joseph Rowntree Foundation.

Willcocks, D., Peace, S. and Kellaher, L. (1987) *Private Lives in Public Places: A Research Based Critique of Residential Care in Local Authority Old People's Homes*. London: Tavistock.

Williams, F. (1989) *Social Policy: A Critical Introduction – Issues of Race, Gender and Class*. Cambridge: Polity.

Williams, F., Popay, J. and Oakley, A (eds) (1999) *Welfare Research: A Critical Review*. London: UCL Press.

Wilson, G. (1991) Models of ageing and their relation to policy formation and service provision, *Policy and Politics*, 19(1): 37–47.

Wilson, G. (1997) A post modern approach to structured dependency theory, *Journal of Social Policy*, 26(3): 341–50.

Wilson, D., Aspinall, P. and Murie, A. (1995) *Factors Influencing Housing Satisfaction among Older People*. Birmingham: Centre for Urban and Regional Studies.

Wiseman, R. (1980) Why older people move, *Research on Ageing*, 2(2): 141–54.

Index

accessibility, 87
Acheson Report, 72
achievements, 57
Acts of Parliament
  Care Standards 2000, 123
  Chronically Sick and Disabled Persons
    1970, 106–7, 109, 117
  Community Care Direct Payments
    1996, 41
  Housing 1996, 46, 152
  Housing Grants, Construction and
    Regeneration 1996, 103, 104,
    110–11
  Local Government and Housing 1989,
    98, 100, 107–9
  National Assistance 1948, 106, 121
  NHS and Community Care 1990, 43,
    63, 82, 107, 121, 126
  Residential Homes 1984, 123, 129
adaptations, 53, 106–14
advocacy, 99, 166
affordability, 134
age, 4, 9–10, 26–30
Age Concern, 15, 111, 131
Age Concern Institute of Gerontology,
  33
ageism, 23–4, 26, 134
allocation, 49
allowances, 14, 125
Alzheimer's disease, 70

Anchor Trust, 65, 66, 98
assessment, 52, 57, 63, 66, 108, 109
assistive technology, 114–15
attendance allowance, 14
Audit Commission, 44, 64, 126
Avon Health Authority, 68, 73

baby boomers, 4
bathing, 111
bathrooms, 56
bereavement, 9, 86–7
Best Value, 139, 145
Better Government for Older People
  initiatives, 15, 141
Better Services for Vulnerable People
  Department of Health, 143
biographical approach, 25
Birmingham, 103
Booth, Charles, 12
boundary issues, 166
*Building Bridges: A Guide to Arrangements
  for Inter-Agency Working*
  (Department of Health), 145, 152
building regulations, 113
buildings, 48

care, 128–31
care allowances, 125
care management, *see* assessment
Care and Repair, 98, 100, 116, 126

Care Standards Act 2000, 123
carers, 54
Caring for People: Community Care in the Next Decade and Beyond (White Paper), 41, 63, 64, 126, 144
Census returns, 14
change, 14
Charity Organization Society (COS), 12, 14, 15
Chronically Sick and Disabled Persons Act (CSDP) 1970, 106–7, 109, 117
chronological age, 4
collaboration, 138
collective living, 118, 119
commodes, 111, 112
common interest developments (CIDs), 8
communal living, 118–36, 131–2
community care, 17, 31, 51, 61–6, 82–3
Community Care Direct Payments Act, 41
complaints, 53
confidentiality, 145, 146, 151
Conservative governments, 144, 151
consumerism, 27, 162
continuity, 14
control, 58
convalescence, 112
cooperation, 138
coordination, 138
Cornwall social services, 52
costs, 86, 116, 166
council housing, 13, 45
councillor perspectives, 52–3
crime, 87

databases, 94
deaths, 58
decline, 25–6
dementia, 70, 71, 123, 130, 142, 146
Denmark, 124
Department of the Environment, Transport and the Regions, 99, 151
Department of Health, 66
dependency, 23, 35, 36, 66
depression, 70, 71, 72
deprivation, 37
difference, 6–10
disability, 28, 106, 108, 117, 140
disability movement, 110, 140–1
disabled facilities grant, 108, 110, 111
discrimination, 109–10, 111, 157

disengagement theory, 22, 30
district councillors, 53
district nurses, 54
diversity, 4
domestic help, *see* home carers
domicilary services, 14, 62, 123

Elderly Accommodation Council (EAC), 78, 94
elderly person's adaptation grant, 101
emotional issues, 89, 93
empowerment, 25, 93
English House Condition Surveys (EHCS), 97, 116
ethnicity, 5
extreme old age, 9–10

The F Factor (Department of Health), 122
falling, 87
fear, 9, 87, 97
Fife domiciliary services report, 51–2
finance, 86, 89, 105–6
fitness standard, 105
front line workers, 54
funding, 63, 99, 124
future needs, 50

general practitioners (GPs), 68
gerontology, 24–5, 30
government perspective, 42–7
grandparenthood, 7–8
grants
    disabled facilities, 108, 110, 111
    elderly person's adaptation, 101
    and home improvement agencies, 99
    housing, 103
    proposed changes, 105
    renovation and repair, 100–6
    Staying Put, 101
Green Papers
    Housing, 45, 46, 49, 105
    Our Healthier Nation, 67
Griffiths Report, 63, 64, 144
Gulliver's Travels J. Swift, 10

Hartrigg Oaks, 88
health, 8–9, 67–73
Health Action Zones, 73, 142
Help the Aged, 15, 57
high-rise housing, 48
Hill, Octavia, 12, 15

historical perspective, 10–14
home, 3, 30–4, 57–8, 120
Home Alone Audit Commission, 126
home carers, 51, 54, 56, 57
Home Energy Efficiency Scheme, 106
home improvement, 67, 105
home improvement agencies (HIAs), 54,
    64, 65, 98–100
home ownership, 33
home repairs assistance(minor works
    assistance), 101–2, 103
homelessness, 2–3, 5, 71–2
HOOP (Housing Options for Older
    People) project, 56, 59, 78, 90–4
hospital discharge, 112–13
hotel model, 36
household composition, 14
housing, 3, 39
    and community care, 64–6
    and health, 67–74
    and joint working, 145, 149
    older people's perspective, 56, 81–2
    see also sheltered housing; very
    sheltered housing
Housing Act 1996, 46, 152
housing associations, 65, 73, 131, 146
housing benefit, 45–7, 160
housing conditions, 97–8
housing design, 87, 115
housing equity, 162
housing grants, 103
Housing Grants, Construction and
    Regeneration Act 1996, 103, 104,
    110–11
Housing (Green Paper) (DETR), 45, 46,
    49, 105
housing manager, 50
housing officers, 54
housing options, 78
Housing Options for Older People
    (HOOP) project, 56, 59, 78, 90–4
housing status, 5
housing stock, 48
humanistic perspective, 25

identity, 26, 27–8
illness, 69–70
immigrants, 84
impairment, 140
improvement, 50
income, 4, 86, 97, 98, 129
independence, 55–7, 90, 96–117

independent living, 35, 36, 41, 130–1,
    157
independent sector, 63
indifference, 97–8
individuals, 22
information, 145, 152
institutions, 120, 131, 134
inter-agency working, *see* joint working
involvement, 164

Japan, 43
joined up thinking, 42, 142–4
joint working, 138, 139–42, 144, 145–8,
    166–7
Joseph Rowntree Foundation, 65, 88,
    113

Labour government, 15, 151
Last Refuge, The Townsend, P., 124
later life, 2–3
legacies, 59–60
leisure, 7
lifetime homes, 50, 113–14, 130
life experience, 6
*Living Independently: A Study of the
    Housing Needs of Elderly and Disabled
    People*, 35, 36, 37
local authorities, 63, 99
local authority homes, 121, 123
Local Government and Housing Act
    1989, 98, 100, 107–9
local perspectives, 47–53
loneliness, 58–9, 88

*Making Partnerships Work in Community
    Care* Means, R. *et al.*, 137, 148–53
managers, 50, 50–2
mental health, 71, 72
mind set, 163–4
minor works assistance (home repairs
    assistance), 101–2
minority groups, 8, 71, 84, 93
mixed economy, 65
mobility, 34, 87
Modernising Social Services (White Paper),
    66, 105, 128
mortality, 9
moving, 77–95, 85–6

National Assistance Act 1948, 106, 121
National Care Standards Commission,
    123

National Federation of Housing
  Associations (NFHA), 65, 73
national insurance, 13
National Preventive Task Group, 66
neighbourhoods, 88
Netherlands, 42, 113, 134
networks, 139
Newcastle-upon-Tyne, 143
NHS and Community Care Act 1990, 43,
  63, 82, 107, 121, 126
Norway, 77
nursing homes, 63, 64

occupational therapists, 54, 108, 113
old age, 26–30
Ombudsman, 109
Our Healthier Nation: A Contract for Health
  (Green Paper), 67

partnerships, 139, 143, 146, 148–54
Partnerships in Action (Department of
  Health), 138, 143
pensions, 12, 13, 14
personal issues, 89
phenomenological perspective, 25
planning, 50
policy, 15, 34–9, 41, 49, 156–67
policy action teams, 142
political economy approach, 23, 24, 25
population, 13
postmodern society, 26, 27, 28, 33
postwar period, 12–14
preventive agenda, 65, 66, 105, 165–6
primary care, 67
privatization, 27, 28
professionals, 147, 149
providers, 41
public spending, 45–7
pull factors, 89–90
push factors, 86–8

Quality and Choice: A Decent Home for All
  (DETR), 165

RADAR (Royal Association for Disability
  and Rehabilitation), 111
regeneration, 142, 143
registration, 130
rehabilitation, 112
relatives, 132, 134
renovation, 100–6
renovation and repair grants, 100–6

repair/disrepair, 50, 96–8, 100–6, 101–2
reports, 51–2, 63, 64, 72, 144
research, 32–3, 163
residential care, 23, 63, 64, 119, 121,
  128, 131
Residential Homes Act (RHA), 123, 129
resourcing, 154
retirement, 83–4, 88
right to buy, 48
Royal Association for Disability and
  Rehabilitation (RADAR), 111
rural settings, 5

Saving Lives: Our Healthier Nation (White
  Paper), 67, 73
Scottish Office, 44
Seaside and Country Homes Agency, 83
self, 57–8, 120
service commissioning, 138
service delivery, 60
service provision, 138
sheltered housing, 13, 82, 120, 124–7
  and dementia, 71
  potential, 65
  reasons for moving into, 56
  and special needs, 37
  see also very sheltered housing
shortage, 45
single regeneration budget (SRB), 142
Smart houses, 114
social construction, 23, 30
social exclusion, 140
social inclusion, 106, 156, 165
social services, 50–2, 68, 107, 113
  and joint working, 146, 150
special needs, 37–8, 126
spending cuts, 52
stakeholders, 151
state provision, 12
status, 85
Staying Put, 65, 82, 98, 100, 101
stereotypes, 146–7
strategic planning, 138
subsidies, 63
support services, 45–7, 66
supported housing, *see* special needs
Supporting People (DSS), 47, 66, 99, 127,
  159, 166
Swift, J. *Gulliver's Travels*, 10

technology, *see* assistive technology
tenure, 33–4, 111, 126, 162

Test of Resources, 108, 109, 110
theoretical perspectives, 22–30, 38
tolerance, 97–8
Townsend, P. *The Last Refuge*, 124
transfer, 49

under-occupation, 45
underfunding, *see* funding
United States, 8, 42
urban settings, 5
users, 41

vertical warden schemes, 48
very sheltered housing, 125, 128–34
vulnerability, 5, 41

Wales, 53, 80, 99, 100, 102

wardens, 48, 54, 127, 146
wealth, 4
websites, 94
welfare state, 12, 27
White Papers
   *Caring for People: Community Care in the
     Next Decade and Beyond*, 41, 63, 64,
     126, 144
   Modernising Social Services, 66, 105, 128
   Saving Lives: Our Healthier Nation, 67,
     73
With Respect to Old Age (Royal
   Commission) (NHS Confederation),
   64, 115, 123, 128, 131, 166
workshops, 153

York, 88

UNDERSTANDING OLDER HOMELESS PEOPLE

Maureen Crane

This is a remarkable book, based on Maureen Crane's many years of acquaintance with homeless people. It throws light on the pathways which lead to homelessness, and should be required reading not only for policy makers in this field, but all those interested in the vicissitudes of the human life course.

Peter G. Coleman, Professor of Psychogerontology,
University of Southampton, UK

Drawing on 10 years' experience of working with the elderly homeless, Maureen Crane has produced a book that will be of immense value to those who wish to understand more about this growing social problem.

Bryan Lipmann, Victoria, Australia

This book is destined to become the standard reference for anyone interested in ageing and homelessness.

Carl I. Cohen, Professor, Department of Psychiatry,
State University of New York Health Science Center at Brooklyn, USA

Although ageing people are a significant segment of the homeless population, they have largely been ignored by service providers and policy makers. This remarkable book sets out to remedy this situation and offers new research on the causes of homelessness. Partial life histories have been collected from older homeless people and their pathways into homelessness traced. Although the book is about older homeless people, many of them have been homeless since they were teenagers or since early adulthood. It therefore examines the reasons for homelessness at all stages of the life course. The book discusses the circumstances, problems and needs of older homeless people, looks at how services are responding, and makes recommendations for service development. Case studies are used throughout to assist explanations.

This book has much to offer a wide audience including service-providers, policymakers, healthcare workers, housing and social services workers, gerontologists and sociologists. Because it is easy to read, it is accessible to lay readers. It will be of interest to a British audience and an international audience, particularly in countries such as America and Australia where innovations in services for homeless older people are rapidly developing.

Contents
Studying older homeless people and their needs – Homelessness: a history of concepts and theories – Part I: Biographies and pathways into homelessness – The prevalence and profiles of homelessness among older people – The breakdown of family households – Itinerant working lives – Mental illness and stressful events – The aetiology of homelessness among older people: a synthesis – Part II: Meeting the needs of older homeless people – the circumstance of older homeless people and their problems – British policies and services to address homelessness – Resettling older homeless people – Appendices – References – Index.

224pp   0 335 20186 5 (Paperback)   0 335 20187 3 (Hardback)

HOUSING AND PUBLIC POLICY
CITIZENSHIP, CHOICE AND CONTROL

Alex Marsh and David Mullins (eds)

- Is change in housing driven by policy or by wider social and economic factors?
- How have policy changes affected citizens' rights to housing?
- What has been the impact of housing policy on the choices available to producers and consumers and the control over housing consumption and production?

This book is designed for readers who require an up-to-date and relevant account of housing policy and are interested in the relationship between housing policy and wider social change. Recent policy changes are described, drawing on leading-edge research by the authors, and interpreted using an innovative framework incorporating the concepts of citizenship, choice and control. This approach allows housing studies to be linked with broader issues, and to adopt a questioning approach to distinguish rhetoric from reality in the policy process. While individual chapters provide accessible accounts of change occurring in the specific tenures (owner occupation, private renting, local authorities and registered social landlords), the book as a whole provides a broader overall picture in which these changes can be understood. In particular the authors trace the development and impact of contested ideas of social rights and citizenship on access to and control of housing. The focus on housing policy in Britain in the 1980s and 1990s is widened by considering examples of the different ways citizenship has been constructed in other societies and over a longer period of time.

Contents
Processes of change in housing and public policy – Differentiated citizenship and housing experience – Housing policy, citizenship and social exclusion – Secure and contented citizens? Home ownership in Britain – Expanding private renting: flexibility at a price? – More choice in social rented housing? – Incentives, choice and control in the finance of council housing – A prize of citizenship? Changing access to social housing – Charters in housing: enhancing citizenship, promoting choice or reinforcing control? – More control and choice for users? Involving tenants in social housing management – Rhetoric and reality in housing policy – Index.

272pp   0 335 19925 9 (Paperback)   0 335 19926 7 (Hardback)

THE MATURE IMAGINATION
DYNAMICS OF IDENTITY IN MIDLIFE AND BEYOND

Simon Biggs

- What does it mean to possess a mature imagination under contemporary social conditions?
- Is it possible to choose not to grow old?
- How are the core questions for adult identity to be addressed in midlife and beyond?

This innovative and wide-ranging book critically assesses notions of adult ageing as they affect people's lifestyles and their sense of personal and social identity. Drawing on an extraordinary range of theory, original research and empirical sources, Simon Biggs examines the interpretation of these changes within social theory and their implications for practice in therapy and in health and welfare settings.

Biggs' argument develops a number of key concepts, and begins by assessing notions of change arising from psychodynamic and postmodern perspectives on ageing. Whilst these ideas shape our understanding, the study of ageing itself challenges easy theoretical assumptions about adult identity. The author critically assesses the contribution of these key perspectives and develops a model for combining the inner world of the mature imagination with the possibilities and uncertainties inherent in contemporary social life. Central to this analysis are tensions between authenticity and masquerade, personal coherence and continuity, and the role of facilitative and restrictive social space. The reader is invited to transgress traditional subject boundaries and draw on insights from sociology, psychotherapy and social gerontology in new and creative ways. The issues that emerge are of both theoretical and practical importance and are presented clearly and concisely.

The Mature Imagination should be of interest to a broad range of students and practitioners in the areas of counselling, health and welfare as well as readers interested in following debates in contemporary social theory.

Contents
Introduction – Maturity and its discontents – From ego psychology to the active imagination – Postmodern ageing – Masque and ageing – Midlifestyle – Meaning and forgetting – Social spaces and mature identity – Policy spaces in health and welfare – Conclusions and implications – References – Index.

224pp   0 335 20102 4 (Paperback)   0 335 20103 2 (Hardback)